SW

03.03.08

C.

C

UNDERSTANDING TREATMENT
WITHOUT CONSENT

Understanding Treatment Without Consent

An Analysis of the Work of the Mental Health Act Commission

Edited by

IAN SHAW
University of Nottingham, UK

HUGH MIDDLETON
University of Nottingham, UK

JEFFREY COHEN
Former Head of Policy of the Mental Health Act Commission

ASHGATE

Published by
Ashgate Publishing Limited
Gower House
Croft Road
Aldershot
Hampshire GU11 3HR
England

Ashgate Publishing Company
Suite 420
101 Cherry Street
Burlington, VT 05401-4405
USA

Ashgate website: http://www.ashgate.com

British Library Cataloguing in Publication Data
Shaw, Ian
    Understanding treatment without consent : an analysis of
    the work of the Mental Health Act Commission
    1. Great Britain. Mental Health Act Commission 2. Great
    Britain. Mental Health Act 3. Mental health services -
    Great Britain 4. Mental health services - Great Britain -
    History
    I. Title II. Middleton, Hugh III. Cohen, Jeffrey
    362.2'0941

Library of Congress Cataloging-in-Publication Data
Shaw, Ian, 1957-
    Understanding treatment without consent : an analysis of the work of the Mental
Health Act Commission / by Ian Shaw, Hugh Middleton, and Jeffrey Cohen.
        p. cm.
    Includes bibliographical references and index.
    ISBN 978-0-7546-1886-7
    1. Involuntary treatment--Law and legislation--England. 2. Mental health laws--
England. 3. Great Britain. Mental Health Act Commission. I. Middleton, Hugh, 1950-
II. Cohen, Jeffrey, 1949- III. Title.
    [DNLM: 1. Great Britain. Mental Health Act Commission. 2. Mental Health Services--
legislation & jurisprudence--Great Britain. 3. Mental Health Services--organization &
administration--Great Britain. 4. Government Agencies--organization &
administration--Great Britain. 5. Health Care Reform--legislation & jurisprudence--
Great Britain. 6. Patient Rights--legislation & jurisprudence--Great Britain. WM 33
FA1 S534u 2007]

    KD3412.S52 2007
    344.4104'4--dc22
                                                                            2007011095

ISBN 978-0-7546-1886-7

Printed and bound in Great Britain by Antony Rowe Ltd, Chippenham, Wiltshire.

Contents

List of Figures and Tables

Introduction

Ian Shaw

We are in an era when choice of and consent to treatment are fundamentally at the centre of the health service modernisation process. This recognises the autonomous right of individuals – with capacity for rational thought – to decide what should and can be done with their own bodies. Such principles are now framed as human and citizenship rights.

The central assumptions underpinning these rights are based upon the individuals' capacity for rational thought. Once it has been decided that the patient is incapable of rational thought and treatment decisions are taken away from them, that person's rights have been removed. That raises a whole set of other issues, in particular the role of psychiatrists and other professionals in making such decisions and the duty of care that flows from it. This is the context of the Mental Health Act Commission's (MHAC) work, ensuring the care and rights of people subjected to the various sections of the Mental Health Act.

This is the context of this book. Its genesis lies in a Department of Health funded research project, which included analysis of the data held by the MHAC. That analysis is included in the pages of this text as are the other issues that arose from the project, which informed the Government's review of the Mental Health Act. However, the book also goes beyond that research project to explore contemporary issues facing the MHAC and the changing context of its work. The book is far more policy oriented than the earlier, and extremely good, socio-legal work on the changing perceptions of consent in mental illness over the last 150 years, written by Phil Fennell (1996). Although very much a jointly authored text, the work in the book does have some recognisable delineation. Ian Shaw has taken the role of lead editor in association with Hugh Middleton. Ian also wrote the introduction, chapter one's short history of mental health, and contributed to chapters three, four and the final chapter. Jeff Cohen wrote the second chapter on the development of the MHAC, the fifth chapter on the process of reform of the Act and much of the final chapter. Hugh Middleton assisted with the editorial task and led contributions on chapter three's review of the work of the Commission and chapter four's review of the work of second opinion appointed doctors. Connor Duggan contributed a significant discussion of the treatability criteria in Psychopathic disorder, illustrating continuing issues in care. Simon Boyes and Michael Gunn also contributed a significant chapter on the Legal aspects of mental health care and the role of the MHAC.

Just 10 years after the passing of the 1983 Mental Health Act, the Mental Health Act Commission, in its Fifth Biennial Report, was urging that a full review of the 1983 Act was required. It was a further six years before the then Secretary of State for Health commissioned an urgent review arguing, "we do not have time to spend in years of contemplation" (DH, 1999). However, the Department of Health has of course done exactly that. A consultation document was released but had such negative feedback that it looks, to all intent and purposes, as if the review has been shelved. This then leads to the final chapter of the book, which is a brief discussion on the changing role of the MHAC and its merger with the Health Care Commission (formally Commission for Health Improvement) by 2008 and the continuing issues that any such organisation would have to contend with. We hope you will find the work of use.

References

Department of Health (1999), *Review of the Expert Committee: Review of the Mental Health Act 1983*, Cm 4480, London.

Fennell, P. (1996), *Treatment Without Consent: Law, Psychiatry and the Treatment of Mentally Disordered People Since 1845*, London: Routledge.

Chapter 1

A Short History of Mental Health

Ian Shaw

Concern for people with mental illness has waxed and waned through the centuries, but the development of modern day approaches to the subject dates from the mid 18th Century. Up until the middle of the 18th Century services for people with mental illness reflected dominant perceptions of the insane at the time. These attitudes came from the increasing influence of reason and rationality on public consciousness. Madness was a form of unreason and therefore had to be controlled. In England it was the workhouse that was used for such confinement until the mid 18th Century.

In 1744 the Vagrancy Act recommended that each English county should be allowed to set up an asylum to which both criminal and pauper lunatics could be sent. Admission decisions were to rest with local Justices rather than physicians. During the early 19th Century the gradual development of County asylums occurred not only without medical influence, but also with a relatively sophisticated non-medical approach termed 'moral treatment'. From this point of view the experience of madness was to be corrected by providing a calm and ordered life, in which the sufferer was treated in so far as possible in a humane and respectful manner. Symbolised by the dramatic removal of the chains of the inmates in 1774 by Pinel in the asylums of Bicêtre and Saltpetrière, this approach was developed by Tuke at the Retreat in York into an educational process, using kindness and respect to help people re-establish self-control of their 'animal natures' through moral force. In "Description of the Retreat" (1813), Tuke argued that a patient's "desire for esteem" rather than "the principle of fear" guided the organisation of treatment.

Partly in response to this example, and partly in reaction to the excesses of private mad-houses revealed in Parliamentary reports in 1807 and 1815, a strong reform movement developed to press for the construction and regulation of public asylums. The construction of these was made compulsory in the 1845 Lunatics Act; within three years nearly three-quarters of English counties had complied, and the rest followed suit within 10 years. While it might be expected that the non-medical system of 'moral treatment' would naturally be adopted in these new asylums, in fact the medical profession soon came to dominate them.

The asylum movement drew its inspiration not only from medicine and moral treatment, but also from the utopian hopes which inspired socialist and religious communards of the early 19th Century, such as Robert Owen. Yet by 1877 a Lancet commission set up to investigate asylums recorded that "everywhere attendants, we are convinced, maltreat, abuse and terrify patients when the backs of the medical officers are turned" (Jones, 1972). The asylums had rapidly become overcrowded during the middle of the century as a result both of pressure on them to take increasing numbers, and the failure of the asylum doctors to cure their inmates. At the end of the first quarter of the 19th Century there were six public asylums with an average size of 116 beds; by 1850 this had grown to 24 asylums averaging 300 beds, and by 1880 it was 60 asylums averaging 650 beds each (Scull, 1979, p.198).

By the early 1900s public asylums were thus widespread. However, these were not run on the principles envisaged by the reformers. The overwhelming feature of the new public asylums was their custodial role. This was partly a reflection of their original design. In Britain, the 1808 Lunatics Act stated:

> All lunatics, insane persons or dangerous idiots, so committed to such asylums, shall be safely kept ... no such person shall be suffered to quit the asylum or be kept at large until the visiting justices, or the greater part of them shall order the discharge of such persona. (Busfield, 1986)

However, the management of these public asylums of rapidly increasing size further added to their custodial nature and reflected the view of government and society about the need to control madness. A regimented routine and the creation of passivity and dependence in inmates enabled a system of strict control. A writer in 1859 commented:

> In a colossal refuge for the insane, a patient may be said to lose his individuality and to become a member of a machine so put together as to move with precise regularity and invariable routine; – a triumph of skill adapted to show how such unpromising materials as crazy men and women may be drilled into order and guided by rule, but not as apparatus calculated to restore their pristine condition and their independent self-governing existence. (on the state of lunacy and the legal provision for the insane, with observations on the construction and organisation of asylums, 1859)

The ultimate symbol of this desire for efficient control was the Panopticon, invented by Jeremy Bentham in 1843 (Figure 1.1).

The Panopticon, in Foucault's terms (1965), extended the 'gaze' of the observer, such that in principle one person, at the centre, could maintain a large number of inmates under surveillance simultaneously. Indeed through the careful use of screens, it would become impossible for inmates to know when they were actually under surveillance, and hence the observer could maintain the effect of continuous observation even in their absence.

Although there were renewed efforts to introduce therapeutic regimes into British asylums towards the end of the 19th Century the 1890 Lunacy Act concentrated more on protecting the rights of the public outside of the asylum. It did this by tightening up the legal procedures that could lead to detention. Jones views this Act as a 'triumph of legalism' in that the power of the legal profession had overcome the power of the medical and social policies of the time. The implications of this were to hamper the progress of the mental health movement for nearly 70 years:

> The movement for further reform of the law became an (unequal) affair of pressure groups. The legal profession had been fully established for centuries. Medicine was involved in throwing off the shackles of a long association with barbering and charlatanism, and did not achieve full status until the passing of the Medical Registration Act of 1858 ... social

work and social therapy were to remain occupations for the compassionate amateur until well into the twentieth century. It is therefore not surprising that the legal approach took precedence, to be followed after 1890 by the medical approach. It is only now, when the social sciences have developed a comparable professional status that the social approach is coming into its own again. (Jones, 1961)

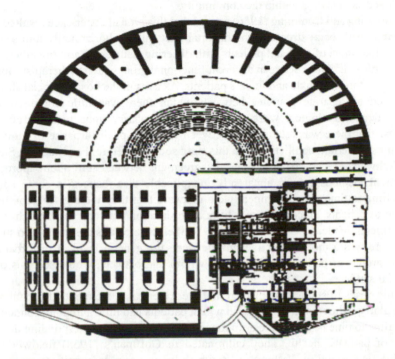

Figure 1.1 The Panopticon

Asylums – Critiques and Alternatives

There have been two major policy objectives of reformers over the last century. The first of these was to reform the asylums, and the second to replace them. The reform of the custodial asylums into 'proper' hospitals was initiated in Britain by the Mental Treatment Act of 1930 that moved the focus away from detention and towards prevention and treatment (Busfield, 1986), and stimulated the introduction of insulin coma therapy, electro-convulsive therapy, and brain surgery. The experience of 'shell-shock' during the First World War had dramatically illustrated the way in which healthy people could succumb to mental distress. During the 1940s and early 1950s there was also a growing humanitarian critique in America of the institutional regime that had developed in the asylums. Important early works included those of Bateman and Dunham (1948) and Belknap (1956) on the American State mental hospital. These authors disregarded the medical view of hospital life in favour of viewing mental hospitals in terms of human communities. Many mental hospitals were situated in rural settings and provided the majority of local workers with employment. Jobs were 'spoken for' from generation to generation within families, who frequently lived in or near the hospital site. Traditional and routine approaches to nursing work became very stable, and difficult to change. Their findings pointed to the existence of a rigidly stratified human community. Patients at the bottom of a hierarchy of power were thus unable, either individually or collectively, to press their needs and claims within the community.

Cumming and Cumming (1956) argued that this typical experience resulted from a 'granulated' social structure: the hospital was split up horizontally into separate 'caste'-like strata of staff and patients with differing statuses. In addition, there were rigid vertical divisions between different functional groups such as therapists, nurses, administrators, and male and female patients. As a result the hospital social structure consisted of separate granules between which there was little communication. Detailed anthropological work developed these observations more carefully to suggest that there was relationship between the level of disturbance of individual patients and certain conflicts within this rigid social structure. For example, Stanton and Schwartz (1954) suggested that disagreement between staff about appropriate treatment methods caused apparently inexplicable disturbances in some patients from time to time. Staff members were unaware that they were giving conflicting advice to patients, since there was little co-ordination between working shifts and departments. Miller (1957) and Caudill (1958) elaborated this observation to suggest that there was a more collective link between the general level of disturbance in whole groups of patients, and conflicts within and between whole sections of the medical staff.

This series of studies established that the American State mental hospital was a particularly static routinised place, in which patients had little autonomy, punctuated from time to time by explosive eruptions of tension, and the corresponding deterioration of patients' health. They culminated in Goffman's (1958) fieldwork in a psychiatric hospital in Washington, in which he proposed to classify them as 'total institutions', causing palpable damage to patients through the 'mortification of self' in a 'moral career' from human being to inmate. This work, followed by a series of hospital enquiries and research findings throughout the early 1970s led first to the favouring of 'therapeutic communities' to improve conditions in mental hospitals and then care in the community emerged as the main policy option.

This was the second policy objective to emerge after the 1930 Act, which became more widely accepted after the Second World War: to move the locus of treatment away from the asylums altogether by developing broad systems of community care. The 1930 Act had given the local authorities permissive responsibilities for the aftercare of those discharged from hospital though it was not until the 'three revolutions' of the 1950s (Jones, 1975) that a significant move towards community care occurred. The first 'revolution' was the introduction of new drugs. Clorpromazine (largactil), although sedative in effect, enabled that patient to continue daily activities whilst being relieved of the more disturbing symptoms of their illness. The second 'revolution' was an administrative one which involved the modernisation of hospitals to utilise a wide range of services – such as: inpatient, outpatient units; day care; hostels etc – this facilitated the development of community care. The third 'revolution' involved legal reforms brought about by the Mental Health Act of

1959. This abolished compulsory admission as the regular means of admission and aimed to reorientate the mental health service away from institutional care towards community care.

The reason for these changes in policy away from hospital provision has been the subject of vigorous debate – a debate that echoes wider discussions about how and why welfare systems have developed and changed since the 19th Century. In this case the notion that first medical and then social enlightenment have resulted in policy change, as implied in the previous quote from Kathleen Jones, has been strongly challenged by Andrew Scull. Although Scull recognises the contribution of these developments to the moves towards community care, he does not consider it a sufficient explanation for policy development. Scull also questions the positive interpretation given to the shift towards community care and suggests that economic policies underlined the process. In the early to mid 19th Century the institutionalisation of those who were unable to survive the rigours of wage labour that had spread across the country was the most effective means for governments to cope with them. The building and staffing of asylums was the cheapest solution. Later the establishment of welfare states with national income support systems meant that support in the community could replace more expensive institutionalisation, and the hospitals began to empty well before the 'revolutions' described by Jones. Thereafter, Scull suggests that mental health policy has been driven by the relative costs of alternative technologies of social control, since the medical profession had, and still has, relatively little treatment available: "Segregative modes of social control became, in relative terms, far more costly and difficult to justify" (Scull, 1977, ch.5). Research by Knapp (1999), however, suggests that community care has not had the cost advantages that Scull assumes. Controlling for the quality of care, it appears that community care is not cheaper than hospital care; rather it has been cheaper because the quality of care has been lower. In addition the control function of community care has had some spectacular failures, discussed later, which have now stimulated a major policy review in the UK.

Problems with Community Care

By the mid 1950s there was a downward trend in many countries in the number of patients in mental hospitals. The anti-institutional or de-hospitalisation movement was reinforced by a series of reports of hospital scandals (Martin, 1985) and community care policy became the policy objective of many western countries.

Care of the mentally ill has changed dramatically in the decades since the 1960s. Drugs introduced in the mid 1950s, along with other improved drugs and treatment methods, have enabled many patients who would once have spent years in mental institutions to be treated in the community instead. Treatment of patients with less severe mental disorders has also changed markedly. Previously, patients with mild depression, anxiety disorders and other types of neurosis may have been treated individually with psychotherapy, if they were lucky, or more often with addictive tranquillisers. Although this treatment form is still used, alternative approaches are now widely available. In some instances a group of patients meets to work through problems with the guidance of a therapist; in others families are treated as a unit. As in serious mental illness, the treatment of milder forms of anxiety and depression have been furthered by the introduction of new, less addictive, drugs, such as Prozac, that help to alleviate symptoms.

The few remaining mental hospitals in much of Europe now give complete freedom of buildings and grounds and, in some cases, visits to nearby communities. The most dramatic example is provided by Italy where the mental hospitals were emptied in a short space of time by law. But America, too, has had a vigorous community mental health movement, and declining hospital bed numbers. In both cases, there have been concerns that the community care alternative has not been adequate. In the US, community mental health facilities have not been able to compensate for the poverty that all marginalised groups face as well as the hostility from suburban dwellers who support community services in principle, but "not on our street" (Dear and Taylor, 1982). As a result mentally ill people have become concentrated in inner city areas living in very poor circumstances, and often homeless, in what in effect are 'asylums without walls'.

In the UK similar concerns have now surfaced. The release of large numbers of patients from mental hospitals has caused significant problems both for patients and for the communities that become their new homes. Adequate community services often are unavailable to former mental patients, a large percentage of whom do not receive services to meet their needs, or lose contact with services altogether. This was particularly highlighted by the case of Ben Silcock, who climbed into the lions' den at London Zoo, and Christopher Clunis, who stabbed to death Johnathan Zito in the London Underground. Such incidents have been well publicised and have placed a great deal of pressure on the government to ensure that public safety is not compromised by care in the community programmes. This has led to further changes in policy designed to reassert control over people with severe mental illness. There has been a general concern, backed by research (Kagan, 1984) about maintaining quality through a time of organisational change. Supervision registers had been introduced early in 1994 for clients who were deemed to be at risk of harming themselves or others, and the wellbeing of patients on these lists was monitored regularly by care staff. It seemed to the public and government that the registers alone were insufficient.

The Mental Health (Patients in the Community) Bill was implemented in the UK on 1st April 1996. Under this Bill, a patient subject to supervised discharge will be required to abide by the terms of a care plan. The appointed key worker has powers to: require the patient to reside in a particular place; require the patient to attend for medical treatment and rehabilitation; convey a patient to a place where he or she is to attend for treatment. If a patient does not comply with the conditions, the individual's case would be reviewed including the possible need for compulsory admission to hospital. However, key workers have been reluctant to exercise such powers as it threatens the relationship that the professional has built up with the client and the therapeutic benefits gained.

Fear of violence can lead to alarmist or reactive policy making where it becomes linked to a wider modern fear of 'risks' in the context of current economic and social change. Beck (1992) has argued that modern societies are 'risk' societies. Certainly there is widespread fear of crime, for example, often amongst those for whom it is actually the least likely (Hale and Hael, 1984). The media presentation of mental health issues has not helped in this respect (Philo et al., 1997), with a less than accurate presentation of the realities of mental illness. Sensational news about occasional violence committed by patients in the community may become the natural successor to the earlier series of sensational revelations about mental hospital malpractice reviewed by Martin (1985), driving policy on the basis of very short term concerns.

The failure of community care policies for those people with severe mental illness has been officially recognised by the UK Government:

> Care in the community has failed. Discharging people from institutions has brought benefits to some. But it has left many vulnerable patients trying to cope on their own. Others have been left to become a danger to themselves and a nuisance to others. Too many confused and sick people have been left wandering the streets and sleeping rough. A small but significant minority have become a danger to the public as well as themselves. (Frank Dobson, 1998)

The UK Government has undertaken a fundamental review of the Mental Health Acts to include possible measures such as compliance orders and community treatment orders to provide effective and prompt supervised care if patients do not take medication or if their condition deteriorates. Enhanced services are to include an increase in the number of acute mental health beds. There is also to be an emphasis on improving the mental health training for GPs and others in primary health care. This is to be backed by extra funds for mental health services. The intention, in 1998, was then to announce a new mental health strategy to Parliament. However, at the time of writing (March 2004) this has not yet happened. A consultative document was circulated in 2002 (DH, 2002) but was not well received by user groups or health care professionals. The reforms now look unlikely this side of the next general election.

In balancing the scales between the freedom of patients and the control of patients for their own and the public's benefit, this new strategy is likely to increase the legal, physical and financial resources available for social and medical control. The question is what the 'technologies of control' should be. Whatever their humanitarian shortcomings, there is no doubt that the old asylums were effective in terms of control. Is there a way of recapturing that function, while retaining a humanitarian and therapeutic input?

Conclusion

We are in a period of significant social and political change. The UK is witnessing a transformation of the 'welfare settlement' of the 1940s with heated debates about the ideological and moral underpinnings for these developments. New inequalities have arisen which the New Labour Government has committed itself to tackle. Within the mental health services, inequalities have a long history: class, race and gender inequalities have permeated the diagnosis and treatment of mental illness. Caught between the basic concerns to balance social control with care and treatment under conditions of expenditure restraint, these inequalities have often been overlooked, but are nevertheless fundamental features of the mental health services which have significant implications for service quality and effectiveness.

Profound changes are underway in the social and political relationships of care, particularly between lay people and the caring professions, leading to a questioning of the nature of expertise. This is not confined to the UK; there is in many countries a renewed commitment to address inequalities in the experience of health and access to care, alongside growing public and political concerns about the 'risks' attaching to community mental health care. These trends have significant implications for the future of policy and practice in mental health as well as the ways in which those rules are overseen.

References

Bateman, J.F. and Dunham, H. (1948), 'The state mental hospital as a specialised community experience', *American Journal of Psychiatry*, 103, pp.445-448.

Beck, U. (1992), [Risikogesellschaft: auf dem Weg in eine andere Moderne], *Risk society: towards a new modernity*, Sage Publications, London.

Belknap, I. (1956), *Human Problems of a State Mental Hospital*, McGraw-Hill, New York.

Bentham (1843), *Works,* Bowring iv, London.

Busfield, J. (1986), *Managing Madness: Changing Ideas and Practice*, Hutchinson, London.

Caudill, W. (1958), *The Psychiatric Hospital as a Small Society*, Harvard University Press, Cambridge, Mass.

Cumming, J. and Cumming, E. (1956), 'The locus of power in the large mental hospital', *Psychiatry*, 19, pp.126-142.

Dear, M. and Taylor, S.M. (1982), *Not On Our Street: Community Attitudes to Mental Health Care*, Pion, London.

Department of Health (2002), *Mental Health Bill: Consultative Document*, Cm 5538-III, HSMO, London.

Dobson, F. (1998), *Frank Dobson Outlines Third Way for Mental Health*, Department of Health Press Release 98/311, 29th July.

Foucault, M. (1965), *Madness and Civilisation*, Random House, New York.

Goffman, E. (1958), 'Report on a study of St. Elizabeth's Hospital, Washington' in *Symposium on Preventative and Social Psychiatry*, Walter Reed Army Institute of Research, US Government Printing Office.

Hale, B. and Hael, B. (1984), *Mental Health Law*, Sweet & Maxwell, London.

Jones, K. (1961), *Mental Health and Social Policy 1845-1959*, Routledge and Kegan Paul, London.

Jones, K. (1972), *A History of the Mental Health Services*, Routledge and Kegan Paul, London.

Jones, K. (1975), *Mental Health and Social Policy*, Routledge and Kegan Paul, London.

Kagan, R. (1984), 'Organisational Change and Quality Assurance in a Psychiatric Setting', *Quality Review Bulletin*, 9, pp.269-299.

Knapp, M., Hallam, A., Beecham, J. and Baines, B. (1999), 'Private, Voluntary or Public? Comparative Cost Effectiveness in Community Mental Health Care', *Policy and Politics*, Vol. 27(1), pp.25-42.

Martin, J.P. (1985), *Hospitals in Trouble*, Blackwell, Oxford.

Miller, D.H. (1957), 'The aetiology of an outbreak of delinquency in a group of hospitalised adolescents' in Greenblatt, M., Levinson, D. and Williams, R. (eds.) *The Patient and the Mental Hospital*, Free Press, New York.

Philo, G. et al. (1997), 'Media Images of Mental Distress' in Heller, T., Reynolds, J., Gomm, R., Muston, R. and Pattison, S., *Mental Health Matters*, Macmillan Press, London.

Scull, A.T. (1979), *Decarceration: Community Treatment and the Deviant – a Radical View*, Prentice Hall, Englewood Cliffs.

Stanton, A. and Schwartz, M. (1954), *The Mental Hospital*, Basic Books, New York.

Tuke, S. (1813), *Description of the Retreat*, York.

Chapter 2

Tracing the Development of the Mental Health Act Commission and its Predecessors

Jeffrey Cohen

Introduction

The Lunacy Commission, established in 1845, was the first national body set up to oversee the conditions in which people have been detained for reasons of mental disorder. It was succeeded by the Board of Control in 1913, which existed until 1959. There was no watchdog body from 1959 until 1983, when the Mental Health Act Commission (MHAC) was established. Each of these bodies has been required to report to the Secretary of State on an annual, or in the case of the MHAC, on a biennial basis. Much of the content of this chapter has been extracted from those reports.

Every generation assumes that current arrangements and practice are an improvement on what went before. However, while the techniques of care and treatment and the style of service delivery has changed considerably, it is striking how often the same concerns re-emerge in the Reports. The comments made by Viscountess Ruth Runciman, in the Chairman's foreword to the MHAC's Seventh Biennial Report, 1995-97, could have been made by Lord Shaftesbury of the Lunacy Commission:

> ... of growing concern to the Commission is the variation between units in the standard of the care which detained patients are receiving. Members of the Commission are seeing too many wards where staff interaction with patients is minimal, where very little structured activity takes place, where treatment plans ... are more a matter of form than substance and where patients face endless barren days with the administration of medicine as the main therapeutic component of their day.

Commissioners were just as likely to record their dismay at the continuing poor conditions, sometimes degenerating into punitive regimes, in the year 2000 as they were 150 years before. On the other hand, the Lunacy Commission in its final Report of 1913 can point to the

> very material amelioration in the well-being and comfort of the certified insane, in the conditions under which they live, and in the character of the accommodation provided for them. That this result has been largely due to the personal visitation and supervision of the

Commissioners in Lunacy is indisputable. (Sixty-Eighth Report of the Commissioners in Lunacy, p.4)

This Report goes on to decry "the stigma attached to insanity" and to highlight the need for early intervention without "full certification" and for increased funding for "patients on trial" (aftercare). If such funding was available, the Report continues, "patients would not be subjected to the trials and difficulties which are so often responsible for a fresh breakdown." These two issues, the threshold for admission and the balance between hospital and community care, remain as relevant today.

The Establishment of the Lunacy Commission

In 1842, the Lunatic Asylums Inspection Act set up an inquiry into the conditions of establishments which catered for 'lunatics' throughout England and Wales. This was carried out by members of the Metropolitan Commission in Lunacy, whose function had been, since the Madhouse Act (1828), to make regular inspections of asylums and madhouses in London. They inspected all the county asylums, of which there were 15, the privately run licensed madhouses and a sample of workhouses and published a comprehensive report which was presented to Parliament in 1844. As might be expected from any such survey, the Metropolitan Commissioners found a wide variation in standards, particularly outside the Metropolitan area. Licensed madhouses ranged from places in which patients could not have been more 'kindly or judiciously treated' to ones where patients were housed in an almost unbelievable state of filth and neglect. Some places used restraint excessively, as in the following extract from the Report, describing a licensed madhouse in West Auckland:

> In the small, cheerless day room of the males, with only one unglazed window, five men were restrained by leg-locks, called hobbles, and two were wearing, in addition, iron handcuffs and fetters from the wrist to the ankle; they were all tranquil. The reason for this coercion was that, without it, they would escape. (1844 Report, p.54)

Following the visit, mechanical restraint was removed from all but one patient "without accident or inconvenience of any kind" (op cit, p.55).

Another major concern was the massive under provision of places in county asylums and the fact that they were being filled with incurable patients, who remained there for life. The majority of 'lunatics' were paupers and the practice was to detain them in the workhouse until they became dangerous or unmanageable and only then to transfer them to the asylum, when it was too late to effect a cure.

The underlying premise of the 1844 Report and the subsequent legislation was the belief that madness was curable if treated early enough in a properly constructed and resourced asylum (Roberts[1]). However, what prompted the drive towards legislation was not so much sympathy for the plight of the 'mad', but a twofold fear of, on the

---

1   Roberts, A. *The Lunacy Commission, a Study of its Origins, Emergence and Character*, website reference: www.mdx.ac.uk/www/study/01.htm.

one hand, 'dangerous lunatics' being let loose in the community and, on the other, the wrongful detention of the sane.

Just as notorious homicides committed by people with a history of mental disorder has stirred public opinion today and prompted the government to propose legislation to deal with the risk (Home Office, 1999[2]), so did events which occurred in the 1840s. One such case was the mistaken murder of Edward Drummond, the private secretary of the Prime Minister, Robert Peel. The assassin, McNaugton (after whom the rules which govern the determination of criminal insanity are named) had, in fact, intended to kill the Prime Minister. McNaughton's defence was that he was under a compulsion to carry out the deed because he was suffering from a delusion of being persecuted by the Tories. He was declared insane and sent to Bedlam. The Lord Chancellor, Lyndhurst, announced in Parliament in 1843 that there was nothing more the law could do to increase public safety after the event, but that consideration would be given to "measures of precaution stronger than those now in existence." It is likely that these measures were incorporated into the Lunacy Bill and that a national desire for greater protection from 'the mad' was one of the motives that led Parliament to pass the 1845 Lunacy Act (Roberts, op cit).

At the same time, there was growing public alarm about individuals being falsely declared insane and unjustly detained. One such case, publicised in a book "The Madhouse System" in 1841, describes how the author, Richard Paternoster, was confined in a madhouse on the representation of his father in an attempt to defraud him of some money. Paternoster's friends notified the police, the Metropolitan Lunacy Commissioners and the press, but it still took six weeks for him to be released. Such was the concern that, in 1845, the Alleged Lunatic's Friend Society was formed "for the protection of the British subject from unjust confinement on the grounds of mental derangement and for the redress of persons so confined" (Jones, 1974[3]). They became an important pressure group for the introduction of greater legal safeguards, culminating in the Lunacy Act of 1890. Many of the same fears have been aroused today by the government proposals for the indeterminate detention of individuals regarded as dangerous as a result of a severe personality disorder (Home Office, op cit).

The lunacy legislation of 1845 consisted of two Acts: the Lunatic Asylums and Pauper Lunatics Act and the Lunatics Act. The former made it mandatory for county authorities to provide asylums to house their lunatic populations. Previous legislation (The County Asylums Act 1808) had recommended that asylums be built to accommodate pauper lunatics, but by 1844 only 15 counties had built them. The Lunatics Act established the Commission for Lunacy. Outside London, responsibility for licensing and overseeing the conditions in which 'lunatics' were kept had belonged to local magistrates. One of the consequences of the lack of any consistent system of inspection was the diverse and unsatisfactory conditions described in the 1844 Report. The remedy, according to its main author, Lord Ashley, was the creation of a

---

2   Home Office Department of Health (1999) *Dangerous People with Severe Personality Disorder*, Proposals for Policy Development.

3   Jones, K. (1974) *A History of the Mental Health Services*, Routledge and Kegan Paul, London.

powerful and permanent national inspectorate, largely modelled on the Metropolitan Commission.

The Commission for Lunacy had duties of inspection covering all establishments, public and private, which housed lunatics. The remit included:

- annual visits by a legal and medical commissioner to each hospital;
- the licensing of private asylums in the Metropolitan area, which were to be visited four times a year;
- each licensed house in the provinces (where the local magistrates retained the licensing function) to be visited twice a year;
- the power to visit single lunatics kept for profit;
- the power to discharge (apart from criminal or chancery cases) after two visits at an interval of seven days;
- the power to visit gaols and workhouses;
- the receipt of notices about all admissions, discharges, escape or transfer within seven days of the occurrence;
- the supervision of the construction and management of the new county asylums, in conjunction with the Home Office;
- the preparation of annual reports for the Lord Chancellor's Office.

Commissioners could visit at any time during the day or night without notice. They were to inquire about each person kept under restraint and to inspect all records.

The Composition of the Lunacy Commission

The Lunacy Commission consisted of six full-time professionals – three physicians and three lawyers with up to five honorary Commissioners, whose main function was to attend Board meetings. The Lunacy Act 1845 specified that the Chairman should be a lay member, presumably to hold the balance of power between the legal and medical professional interests and to avoid the care of the insane being left to any one group of experts. Lord Ashley (later Earl of Shaftesbury) was the natural appointment as Chairman. He was famed for his work in improving the conditions in factories and mines and had been responsible for steering the lunacy legislation through Parliament.

Ashley's perspective on insanity not only determined the way in which the Commission carried out its work but also was most influential in the approach taken by the asylums until the end of the century. He favoured the 'moral treatment' model, which emphasised Victorian values of industry, moderation and piety and of helping 'lunatics' to regain their dignity and self control. He was convinced that a main cause of madness was intemperance and that alcohol consumption was instrumental in 50 per cent of cases. Although these views reflect Victorian morality, there is some resonance with the current concerns about co-morbidity of mental illness and substance misuse (both alcohol and drugs) (Cohen and Williams, 2000[4]).

Ashley was not impressed by the medical profession's claim to expertise, stating on several occasions that a layman could give as good an opinion on the existence of insanity as a doctor (Hervey, 1985,[5] p.104). Consequently, the Commission did not encourage asylum doctors to experiment with new methods of treatment, which became such a prominent feature of its successor body, the Board of Control. On the other hand, Ashley was strongly opposed to a legalistic approach, whose proponents pushed for more stringent admission procedures. He was more concerned about the risk of delaying treatment of a curable case than the danger of unjust detention.

Ashley recognised the importance of the calibre of the Commissioners, writing in his diary, "we must have the best men in every sense of the word, who can speak with authority to the skilful and experienced persons with whom they will always be in contact and sometimes collision" (quoted in Hervey, op cit). This was reflected in the salary. Full time Commissioners were well rewarded financially, receiving £1,500 salary plus expenses. All the six initial appointees and the Secretary to the Board had been Metropolitan Commissioners and, apart from one who resigned after a few months, were to remain in post for a considerable number of years.

Of the three legal Commissioners, Proctor resigned his position in 1861 (having been a Metropolitan Commissioner since 1833); Lutwidge was killed by a patient in 1873 and Campbell retired in 1878. The incident which brought about Lutwidges's death was described in the Commission's Annual Report for that year as follows:

> Mr Lutwidge ... and ... Mr Wilkes had nearly completed the inspection of the establishment ... The Commissioners were leaving one of the wards, when a pauper patient, named William McKave, an inmate of the ward, who had stealthily approached the group, suddenly raised his arm, and with a long nail, sharpened at the end, dealt a blow at Mt Lutwidge's right temple, which penetrated the skull.

McKave had been seeking a transfer to Broadmoor. He was charged with wilful murder, but found not guilty by reason of insanity.

Some of the medical commissioners evidently stayed on beyond their prime. In 1848, the Lancet ran an editorial about Lunacy Commission appointments. One Commissioner, Prichard, a highly regarded psychiatrist and voluminous writer on the subject of insanity, had died. The Lancet was recommending a clean sweep of the medical commissioners, urging the two remaining medical commissioners (Turner and Hume) to resign given their age and health. They were described as "men verging on second childhood, hardly fitted to uphold their profession against the three active lawyers." Turner, in fact, remained in post until 1855 retiring at the age of 82 and Hume lasted until 1857.

---

4   Williams, R. and Cohen, J. (2000) 'Substance Use and Misuse in Psychiatric Wards', *Psychiatric Bulletin*, 24, 43-46.

5   Hervey, N. (1985) 'A Slavish Bowing Down: The Lunacy Commission and the Psychiatric Profession 1845-1860', in Bynum W., Porter R. and Shepherd, M. eds., *The Anatomy of Madness Vol. 1 Institutions and Society*, Tavistock.

The Lancet was lobbying for the position of medical commissioners to be filled by experienced asylum doctors. This, in fact, did happen with the appointment of Samuel Gaskell as Commissioner from 1849 to 1866. He had been the resident superintendent in the Lancaster County Asylum and was well known for his progressive methods. He was against the general use of mechanical restraint. He had also introduced a regime to prevent bed wetting by regular toileting throughout the night, thus allowing the use of decent bedding rather than straw. Gaskell's influence was pronounced. He was described as,

> a remarkably well informed and painstaking official. Proprietors and superintendents who did not look too minutely into the details for themselves were greatly surprised, and not at all pleased, to find the dignified commissioner looking into beds and cupboards, and all manner of uninvestigated places. (Plarr quoted in Roberts, p.18[6])

This attention to detail sometimes led the Commission to being seen as over-intrusive. One superintendent, J. E. Huxley in Kent, saw the centralised authority of the Commission as a "threat to the constitution", arguing that the Commissioners were overstepping their legal powers and that their remit should be confined to supervising the workings of the lunacy law rather than interfering in the day to day management of the asylum. Eventually, in 1863, the Commission forced the resignation of Huxley, complaining of his excessive use of restraint (Fennell, 1996[7]).

Gaskell generally received the support of the medical profession, being one of the founding members of the Association of Medical Officers of Asylums and Hospitals for the Insane. The AMOAHI, formed in 1841, was the forerunner of the Royal College of Psychiatrists. Two-thirds of subsequent appointments of medical commissioners were asylum superintendents. This created a close bond between the Lunacy Commission and the AMOAHI, which became generally supportive of the policies the Commission pursued in the asylums.

More than half of the legal commissioners were first employed as Secretary to the Commission (as this post was invariably filled by a barrister). Legal appointees, without such experience, were likely to be ignorant of lunacy issues. One such appointee, Frere, on being appointed wrote to his relative, Winslow (editor of the Journal of Psychological Medicine and author of a book "Manual of Lunacy"), "Dear Winslow, I have just been appointed a Commissioner in Lunacy. I know nothing about the subject. Send me your book" (quoted in Mellett[8]).

Administrative support to the Lunacy Commissioners was initially provided by the Secretary and two full-time clerks. The volume of business in organising the work of the Commissioners and in keeping up with statistical returns of an increasing asylum population and associated correspondence led to the Secretariat gradually increasing in size so that, in 1877, the clerical staff numbered nine.

---

6   Roberts, A. *Biographies of Medical Lunacy Commissioners 1828-1912*, website reference: www.mdx.ac.uk/www/study/6biom.htm.

7   Fennell, P. (1996) *Treatment without Consent. Law, Psychiatry and the Treatment of Mentally Disordered People Since 1845*, Routledge.

8   Mellett, D. J. (1981) "Bureaucracy and Mental Illness: The Commissioners in Lunacy" 1845-90, *Medical History*, 25, 221-250.

The Work of the Lunacy Commission

Within the first 18 months of the life of the Commission, 107 Board meetings were held, 409 asylums inspected, and 17,748 patients personally examined (First Annual Report). All the certificates of confinement were transmitted to the Commission's office, where they were checked for any irregularities. Notices of death and discharge were also submitted.

The Commission gradually expanded the amount of statistical information it collected in the belief that assembling a registry of all 'lunatics' and the details of their confinement would be of value in advancing knowledge about the care and treatment of the insane. The Commissioners' annual reports became increasingly voluminous. The early Reports were less than 50 pages. In 1879, the main body of the Report was 140 pages with an additional 303 pages of appendices, including policy statements about the construction and management of asylums, copies of reports on institutions visited and statistics about the number, distribution and comparative costs of 'lunatics' (Mellet, op cit).

The amassing of information gave a detailed picture of the state of mental health services at the time, but it is not clear what other purpose it served. The Lunacy Commission itself found it hard to draw any conclusions from the data.

> The statistical information given in our Annual Reports has gradually increased in bulk and importance and we have reason to believe that among those interested in the care and treatment of the insane, and the question of insanity in its various aspects, this portion of our Report is considered to possess much value. At no time however, have we considered it our duty to draw but the most plain and obvious deductions from the figures ... At present we do not feel our recorded experience is sufficiently extensive to warrant many certain conclusions ... and ... conjectures ... would not ... be attended by any public advantage. (Commissioners in Lunacy, Thirteenth Annual Report (1876) quoted in Mellett, op cit)

The Lunacy Commission was also fastidious in its requirements for establishments to keep their own detailed records of key aspects of patient care. This was, in Ashley's view, a means to provide a safeguard against irregular practice. Only through a system of standardised record keeping is it possible to show, as Fennell writes,

> that those with the clinical power to interfere with a person's freedom have addressed themselves to the correct legal criteria and kept within the limits of their powers. This explains why commissioners from 1845 until today have invariably taken a serious view of failures to keep adequate records, from time to time, attracting unfair charges of obsessional bureaucracy. (Fennell, op cit, p.17)

Amending legislation, the Lunacy Asylums Act 1853 introduced more rigorous recording procedures. Medical officers were required to record the use of restraint and seclusion, its means and duration and the reasons for it. Asylums were also obliged to submit their rules for approval by the Commissioners, acting on behalf of the Home Secretary. In 1879, the Lunacy Commission, in an effort to impose national standards, issued a circular, "Precedents of general rules for the government of lunatic asylums pursuant to S.53 of Lunatic Asylums Act 1853", which Fennel has observed might well be regarded as a forerunner of the Code of Practice to the Mental Health Act 1983.

The imposition of what some asylums saw as petty restrictions was intended not so much to interfere with the individual judgement of doctors, but to prevent certain techniques to control disturbed behaviour being used as a punishment or a substitute for more attentive care. However, the dividing line between care and treatment and punishment can often be blurred.

The Commission sought to restrict, if not abolish, mechanical restraint and to minimise the use of seclusion. The Annual Report of 1862 indicated that mechanical restraint, although still used, was employed in very few places and on very few occasions (quoted in Sheppard[9]). However, other techniques were introduced, which were also liable to be abused as a means of restraint rather than treatment. For example, wet packing, in which a patient was tightly wrapped in a wrung out wet sheet, swathed in blankets, and left for an hour or more, was used as a treatment for acute mania. At first, the Lunacy Commission accepted the practice as a medical treatment, but later required that its use be recorded in the medical notes as a mechanical restraint.

Another dubious treatment was cold baths, where the individual was placed in a shower bath and deluged with water as a means of subduing excitement. The Lunacy Commission sought the prosecution of the medical superintendent, Charles Snape, in one case, in 1856, where a 65 year old patient died after being subjected to heavy use of the bath treatment combined with a powerful emetic. However, the Commission lost. The jury dismissed the indictment on the grounds that the medical superintendent had been employing a recognised medical treatment rather than a method of punishment (Fennell, op cit).

The courts are similarly reluctant today to declare even extreme conditions as contravening human rights if they conform to generally accepted psychiatric practice. For example, the isolation of a patient and handcuffing him to a bed for several weeks did not constitute "inhuman and degrading treatment", as it was regarded as a therapeutic necessity because of his extreme aggressiveness.[10] Following the Snape case, the Lunacy Commission conducted a survey about the use of shower baths and concluded in its Eleventh Annual Report that

> the distinction in many cases made between its use as such [a method of treatment], and its use as a moral means of repressing excitement, and of correcting faulty habits, is vague and undefined; and that, as a general rule, sufficient precautions are not taken against its being resorted to as a punishment. (quoted in Fennell, p.29)

Besides insisting on the recording of the use of seclusion, mechanical and other forms of restraint, the Commission issued guidance as part of the 1879 'Precedents' that hospitals should regulate such procedures by only allowing them to be administered with the authority of a doctor. Paradoxically, as Fennell has pointed out, this legitimised them as medical interventions.

---

9   Sheppard, D. *Development of Mental Health Law and Practice*, www.imhl.com/history.htm (accessed 2002).

10   Herczegfalvy vs Austria (1993) 15 EHRR 437.

Mellett has noted the limitations in the ability of the Lunacy Commission to enforce their recommendations. They were unable to impose on workhouses even minimal standards of humane, medically orientated treatment and record keeping that were expected in the asylums. Outside the metropolitan area, the local magistrates retained the power to refuse renewal of licences and the visiting committees to appoint or dismiss medical superintendents. The Commission was dismayed when the visiting committee of the Surrey asylum re-instated Snape following the shower bath case. The Commission made ruthless use of its annual reports to shame institutions into change, but this did not always work, as the following example from the Seventh Annual Report, about the conditions in the Hull Borough Asylum, shows.

> At the next Visit, in July 1850, the Commissioners reported that an additional Supply of Bedding had been provided, but that in other respects the Asylum was in the same unsatisfactory state as before; and in addition … There were no Rules for the Guidance of the Officers and Attendants; that the Diet Table was not printed or strictly adhered to; that the Ventilation of the Rooms was still imperfect, and the Walls required painting and colouring; that there were no Lavatories, no Shutters in the single Rooms, no Waterclosets in the House and that the Privies were very defective …
>
> The Asylum was again visited, in May 1851, by Two Commissioners, who found some few of the Suggestions contained in former Entrees had been adopted; but the whole condition of the Asylum appeared to them to be so defective, that they drew the Attention of the Board to the Subject in a Special Report.

Several more visits were made to no avail. The Commission admitted that it had no means of compelling the Justices of the Borough, who denied the necessity for many of the changes, to adopt the recommendations other than by calling in the assistance of the Secretary of State.

However, there were signs that the Commission was driving home the message that inhuman and degrading treatment should not go unpunished. In 1870, it reported that 122 attendants had been dismissed from asylums, 46 for being violent or rough towards patients. This included two attendants from Lancaster Asylum who were sentenced to seven years penal servitude for manslaughter (Sheppard, op cit).

The Lunacy Act (1890)

According to Kathleen Jones (op cit), each period in the history of mental health services can be analysed in terms of the relative influence of three approaches: 'the social', where the emphasis is on human relations, 'the medical', where it is on physical treatment and 'the legal', where formalised procedures are to the fore. She describes the 1890 Act as the "triumph of legalism".

Shaftesbury was vehemently opposed to making legal procedures too onerous, which, he argued, would result in admission being delayed until symptoms had become so pronounced they would become incurable. Indeed, he resigned as Chairman of the Commission in 1884, so that he could oppose the 'legalistic' Lunacy Amendment Bill in the House of Lords. In June 1885, the Bill was shelved and he consented to resume his office, only to die in October of that year.

Shaftesbury's death removed an obstacle to reform. Public opinion had also been swayed by a series of well-publicised cases of patients being unjustly confined. The existing lunacy legislation, despite the amendments in 1862, which tightened admission procedures, was seen as an inadequate bulwark against the threat to the liberty of the subject. Confidence in the role of the Commission against unjust confinement was also at a low ebb. Both the serious and popular press ("The Times" and "Titbits") carried articles in 1889 which portrayed the Commission as "ineffectual and enjoying too cosy a relationship with those whom it is supposed to regulate" (quoted in Fennell, op cit). At a conference held under the auspices of the Lunacy Law Reform Association, reported in The Times (8 May 1890), the Commission was denounced as "hopelessly effete" and that it should be abolished with its functions devolved to local bodies.

Despite these misgivings, the role of the Commission was reinforced in the 1890 Lunacy Act, alongside a much-strengthened legal framework governing the detention of 'lunatics'. One of the major changes was that private patients, and not just pauper patients, should not be detained without a judicial order from a Justice of the Peace specialising in such reception orders (Roberts, A., op cit). The 1890 Act laid down an elaborate system of documentation and inspection. As in the 1845 Act, the Lunacy Commission was required to send a medical practitioner and barrister to every public asylum and registered subscription hospital at least once a year, to every licensed house in the metropolitan area four times a year and two visits (in addition to local visitation) by a single commissioner to licensed houses outside the metropolitan area. It had to report to the Lord Chancellor every six months on the number of visits and number of patients seen with a detailed report laid before Parliament once a year.

Visits could be made without notice at any hour of day or night. Commissioners were to make detailed enquiries concerning the construction of the building; the classification, occupation and recreation of patients; the admission, discharge and visitation of all patients; the performance of Divine service; and the use or non-use of mechanical restraint. The Commission was required to place a notice about its function in a conspicuous place in the asylum, so that it could be seen by private patients (but not necessarily pauper patients). Correspondence by patients to a Lunacy Commissioner or certain other persons in authority had to be forwarded unopened.

From time to time, over the next 20 years, the Commission issued further directives limiting the type of straitjacket, 'treatment' baths or wet or dry packs, which were permissible, and specifying requirements for medical oversight and observation by an attendant. Similar regulations were issued regarding seclusion, which was defined as the "enforced isolation of a patient by day, between the hours of 7am and 7pm by the closing, by any means whatsoever, of the door of the room in which the patient is." It had to be authorised by a medical officer and the patient periodically observed.

Board of Control 1913-1930

The Mental Deficiency Act (1913) replaced the Lunacy Commission with the Board of Control. The medical and legal members (of which there were now four each) were transferred to the new organisation with the addition of up to four salaried lay members and three non-salaried. A new departure was that at least one of the paid and one of the unpaid Commissioners was to be a woman. Initially, governmental responsibility was transferred back from the Lord Chancellor to the Home Office before coming under the auspices of the newly formed Ministry of Health in 1919. The future chairmen of the Board of Control were all former senior civil servants from that ministry. These organisational changes signalled a shift back from the legal towards the medical approach to mental health and a closer overlap between the treatment of mental with that of physical illness.

The Board of Control was given an extensive remit covering 'mental deficiency' with responsibilities for the 'supervision, protection and control' over 'defectives'; for the supervision of local authorities in the exercise of their powers under the Act and for the certification and inspection of all institutions for 'defectives'. It administered grants to local authorities and voluntary bodies to develop provision for 'mental defectives'. It was directly responsible for establishing and maintaining State institutions for the violent and dangerous. Commissioners kept the power of discharge (although rarely used), except in the case of criminals or 'inebriates', where the consent of the Home Secretary was necessary.

Local authorities were required to set up mental deficiency committees. An early priority of the Board of Control was to ascertain the number of people who were 'mentally defective'. They sent out a circular to all local authorities, but received a mixed response. In 1920, the Local Authorities counted 10,129 'defectives', which was well below what the Board estimated to be the true figure at about 3.55/1,000. In 1927, the total number ascertained was over 60,000, but local authorities only provided accommodation for 5,301 (Jones).

The lack of institutional provision led the Board to recommend what was thought to be a less satisfactory alternative – community care. The Mental Deficiency Act introduced the possibility of supervision in the community in the form of Guardianship, statutory or voluntary supervision. Guardianship was intended for those who were capable of living a protected life in the community and for whom a guardian was available. The Guardian was conferred with powers and duties analogous to a parent of a child under the age of 14. The provision was little used by local authorities, as they thought it was practically useless. The Board urged greater consideration of its use for suitable cases, i.e. those who can be taught to conform to ordinary social requirements, alongside attendance at occupation or industrial centres. Such centres were being rapidly developed by voluntary associations in the 1920s and 1930s. By 1934, the numbers under supervision had increased to:

Guardianship	3,083
Statutory Supervision	33,377
Voluntary Supervision	22,844

The number of people not in institutional care gave rise to fears about their pro-
creation, given beliefs about the inheritance of mental deficiency. It was argued that
sterilisation could be a means of reducing the number of 'defectives' in the longer
term and, in the shorter, lead to savings in the costs of caring, as it would be safer to
release patients from institutional care. The Board of Control received a number of
queries regarding the permissibility of sterilisation. The standard response was that
sterilisation could only be performed, whether or not there was consent, if it was
for the medical welfare of the patient. Any surgeon contemplating an operation was
advised to obtain a second opinion.

In 1934, a departmental committee was set up under the chairmanship of
Lawrence Brock, who was Chairman of the Board of Control, to examine the question
of sterilisation. The Brock Committee recommended that sterilisation should be
legalised, provided there was valid consent from the patient or, if incapable, from
a parent or guardian and that other safeguards were in place, such as two medical
recommendations scrutinised by the Board of Control. However, at a time when
the Nazis were introducing their brutal programme of sterilisation, there was no
prospect for legislation on the subject.

The number and size of the asylums continued to increase, leading to a decline
in standards.

Table 2.1 The Increase of Asylums

Year	No of asylums	Average no of patients
1827	9	116
1850	24	297
1870	50	542
1900	77	961
1930	98	1221

Overcrowded and understaffed, the asylums could only provide institutionalised
care where personal relationships between patients and staff were hardly possible.
Perhaps the nadir was in the 1920s at the time when Dr Montagu Lomax, who had
been an assistant medical officer at Prestwich Asylum, published his book, "The
Experiences of an Asylum Doctor" in 1921. He wrote about an inhumane regime,
poor nutrition, brutal behaviour by medical officers and attendants and a high death
rate. He commented, amongst other deprivations, on the abuse of solitary confinement
in unheated pitch dark cells, mechanical restraints and the administration of large
doses of croton oil (a laxative) as a punitive measure (Harding[11]). Lomax advocated
for more active therapeutic interventions to promote the return of patients to the

---

11 Harding, T. W. (1990) '"Not Worth Powder and Shot" A Reappraisal of Montagu
Lomax's Contribution to Mental Health Reform', *British Journal of Psychiatry*, 156, 180-
187.

community, far reaching changes in asylum management and a complete reform of mental health legislation. The book, well publicised in the press, hit a public nerve. Questions were asked in the House of Commons and the Ministry of Health set up a committee, under the chairmanship of Cyril Cobb, to investigate and report on the charges made by Lomax.

Lomax was strongly condemned by the psychiatric establishment, including the Board of Control. In their evidence submitted to the Cobb Committee, the Board wanted placed on record, "the most emphatic protest against the methods which Dr Lomax had seen fit to adopt in preparation and publishing his book … the charges made were sheer nonsense and gross calumny" (quoted in Jones, 1974, op cit). The Board's stinging attack was obviously to pre-empt criticisms of its own performance in carrying out its watchdog functions. Lomax maintained that the Commissioners were hoodwinked, alleging that the asylum management, warned in advance of their arrival, would stage-manage their visits.

The Cobb Committee accepted the Board of Control's rather than Lomax's version of asylum conditions. However, they recommended that asylums should have no more than a thousand beds and, in future, be constructed on a villa system, allowing smaller and more specialised units to cater for the differing needs and types of patient. Lomax's criticisms were still influential in the longer term, particularly behind the scenes with the Ministry of Health. Relations between the Ministry and the Board of Control were tense, with the former intent on reducing the latter's span of control. In 1924, a Royal Commission on Lunacy and Mental Disorder was set up to inquire into the existing law and administrative machinery for the certification and detention of persons of unsound mind and the extent to which provision should be made for the treatment without certification of persons suffering from mental disorder. One might have expected the Board of Control to welcome this Royal Commission since they had been advocating for the availability of voluntary treatment. However, it was sceptical of the Ministry of Health's motives, writing in its Report of 1924 that the immediate cause of the appointment of the Commission was not its own desire to achieve legislation of a more enlightened type but the

> uneasiness aroused in the public mind by a number of charges, somewhat recklessly made, to the effect that large numbers of sane persons were being detained as insane, that the whole system of lunacy administration was wrong, and that widespread cruelty existed in our public mental hospitals. (quoted in Jones, p.237)

The Royal Commission was indeed sympathetic to Lomax, his evidence taking up 26 printed pages of the final report (Harding, 1990, op cit). It made far-reaching recommendations which were to shape the 1930 Mental Treatment Act. A fundamental premise was that certification should become a last resort in treatment and not a pre-requisite. For Jones,

> The Royal Commission's Report marked a complete denial of the principles of 1890, and a development from the earlier and more enlightened principles of 1845. The legal view of mental illness was no longer acceptable. The medical view was fully endorsed; and the social view was encouraged in the clauses relating to rehabilitation and after-care.

The Board of Control continued to come under fire in the parliamentary debate on the Mental Treatment Bill. One MP described it as "the mysterious and awful Board of Control. People do not know of its name or how to get at it" (Jones, p.248). Despite the threat to abolish the Board and for its functions to be transferred to the Minister direct, the Mental Treatment Act resulted in its expansion. It became a two-tier authority with a central body consisting of a Chairman and five salaried senior Commissioners and 15 assistant commissioners, who were salaried full-time officials and who would take on the visiting function. The central body had to include one legal and two medical members, and at least one Commissioner had to be a woman. The purpose of this body was to make the Board more accessible and available to deal with queries and complaints.

The Mental Treatment Act made provisions for voluntary treatment. A patient could agree to admission by making a written application to the person in charge of any establishment approved by the Board of Control. A voluntary patient had to give 72 hours notice if (s)he intended to discharge him or herself. The Act also introduced the concept of temporary patient for those incapable of consenting to admission. The duration of a temporary order was six months, which could be extended to a maximum of one year with the permission of the Board of Control.

The Board of Control 1930-1959

The admission of voluntary patients created beneficial ripples throughout the hospital system, not least of which was a change in terminology. The term 'lunacy' was removed from the title of the governing legislation (the Mental Treatment Act); a person could hardly agree to be incarcerated in an asylum as a 'lunatic', but instead entered hospital as a patient for care and treatment. More ward doors had to be opened with some patients being free to leave. The question of open and closed doors featured in the Board of Control's Reports, which, in particular, emphasised the benefits of the parole system. Patients could be gradually allowed outside the ward, the hospital, and then have periods on trial leave at home. Indeed the Board, while recognising that occasional mistakes are bound to occur, recommended that it is better to err on the side of giving too much freedom than too little. "Safety First", it wrote in its Twentieth Report (1933), "is not the best motto for mental hospitals."

The Board of Control, perhaps stung by criticisms of the way patients were warehoused in large asylums, strongly promoted better conditions for individual patients. The Board had been urging for a long time to increase patient activities by, for example, the appointment of a special officer for such a purpose. In its Twentieth Report, the Board commented on the importance of variety of occupation which would maintain the patient's interest and was not purely mechanical. A new development which it encouraged was that of musical exercise and dance. Appearance was also seen as important, particularly for women, for whom it recommended "greater variety of clothing and patterns approximating to those worn by normal people." In 1934, it carried out a survey of entertainments and recreations provided in mental hospitals and found that most hospitals had a programme of activities (cinema shows, sports, dancing).

The Lunacy Commission, Board of Control and Mental Health Act Commission have all claimed not to interfere in clinical decisions, but nevertheless have tried to influence practice by monitoring treatments given. Indeed, the Board of Control was criticised by the Cobb Committee (following the Lomax allegations) for not monitoring the level of sedative and laxative medication more closely. Consequently, the Board required hospitals to submit returns of sedative drug use. An analysis of these in the 1930 and 1931 Reports showed wide variation in use between hospitals without any corresponding difference in order and tranquillity. The Board refrained from interpreting these statistics too closely and did not follow up with further inquiry (or, at least, publish any subsequent findings) about these differences as they said they would do (18th Annual Report).

While the Board could or would not evaluate the efficacy of medical treatments, it was keen to ensure that advantage was taken of the latest medical initiatives for the benefit of patients. Even when the benefits were uncertain, the Board was supportive of experimentation, because it, at least, created the impression that hospitals were pro-active in trying to do everything possible to promote recovery, inspiring hope in patients and relatives.

Fennel (1996, op cit) describes the period between 1930 and 1959 as the "age of experimentation." He gives a detailed account of the range of physical treatments designed either to jolt patients out of their disorder or calm them down, so the underlying causes of their disorder can be worked on. The following list gives examples of treatments given:

- treatment for focal infection, resulting in large scale dental extractions
- malarial treatment for general paralysis of the insane (advanced syphilis)
- narcosis (drug induced prolonged sleep)
- insulin coma therapy
- chemically induced shock
- electro-convulsive therapy
- psycho-surgery
- neuroleptic medication

The Board acted as a type of 'clearing house' for research on these treatments. In its annual reports, it included an appendix of abstracts of research carried out in hospitals throughout England and Wales. This part of the Report was larger in volume than the Board's reporting of its own activities. Sometimes, the Board actively encouraged the application of a new treatment. For example, they promoted clinical trials in the inducement of malaria as a treatment of the general paralysis of the insane. However, the Board was mainly concerned with the safe administration of any treatment. For example, it issued a series of circulars about the risks associated with malarial treatment and how it can be safely administered.

The 1946 National Health Service Act stripped the Board of Control of nearly all its functions. From 1948, the Minister of Health took over responsibility for the administration of hospitals and institutions, the licensing of private homes and hospitals for mental disorder and the control of local authority work. Its position as an independent inspectorate was also compromised by being part of the Ministry of

Health and many of its Board members performing functions for the minister and the Board.

There were discussions in the early 1950s to set up a new body independent of the service providers or Ministry of Health, which would have a duty to examine reception documents, exercise residual powers of discharge and deal with complaints of ill-treatment or improper detention (Fennell, ibid). Such changes were overtaken by the appointment of the Royal Commission on the Law relating to Mental Illness and Deficiency (the Percy Commission), which resulted in the Mental Health Act 1959. The Percy Commission, advised by the Board of Control itself, recommended that its functions could be redistributed to other bodies. The scrutiny of documents and the responsibility for the inspection of hospitals were transferred to local health authorities. There was no longer to be any judicial control prior to admission. Where compulsion was deemed necessary, the decision was to be made by professionals, but, following admission, the need for continued detention could be reviewed by the Mental Health Review Tribunal.

The Establishment of the Mental Health Act Commission

During the 1960s and 1970s there was a series of hospital scandals, alleging ill treatment and exposing very poor conditions, particularly on long stay wards. A Yorkshire Television documentary, "The Secret Hospital", reporting on abusive practices within Rampton Hospital, prompted an inquiry, the result of which was the publication of the Boynton Report in 1980. One of the main recommendations of this Report was the establishment of a body to inspect and monitor all institutions where patients were subject to detention under the Mental Health Act (Fennell). Another major concern, which led to calls for changes in the existing legislation, was the lack of clarity about the legal position of doctors to treat detained patients without consent and the lack of any safeguards on the assumption of such powers. In response, the 1983 Mental Health Act did introduce some additional safeguards to limit professional discretion and enhance the rights of detained patients, including the establishment of the Mental Health Act Commission (MHAC) and new consent to treatment provisions.

The essential role of the MHAC is to keep under review the operation of the Mental Health Act 1983 as it relates to the detention of patients. It carries out this role chiefly by visiting hospitals and mental nursing homes providing care and treatment for patients detained under the Act, meeting with detained patients in private, inspecting the records relating to the patient and producing reports of its findings. It can also investigate complaints made by a detained patient (or in certain circumstances, a relative), which have not received a satisfactory response at local level. The MHAC monitors the operation of the consent to treatment safeguards and appoints doctors to give second opinions. It also monitors the operation of the Code of Practice and periodically submits suggestions for changes in subsequent editions of the Code. It publishes a Biennial Report on its work, which is laid before Parliament and may give advice to the Secretary of State on matters which fall within its remit.

The MHAC's role is visitorial. It does not have any specific legal powers to direct that services should implement its recommendations. The following extract from the White Paper preceding the 1983 Act explains some of the founding principles and expectations of the MHAC.

> … the proposed functions of the Commission will be separate to other inspectorate bodies; the Commission will not inspect and report on services in mental illness and mental handicap in hospitals and units in the way that the Health Advisory Service or the Development Team for the Mentally Handicapped do. The Commission's concern will be the particular problems which arise from detention of specific individuals in hospital rather than the general services which affect all mentally ill and mentally handicapped patients … (para. 34)

> … the Commission will appoint SOADs (Second Opinion Appointed Doctors). This will ensure that the opinions are independent and will enable the Commission both to monitor the use of the power to impose treatment and to offer advice on professional and ethical complexities … the Commission will build up considerable expertise in the care and treatment of detained patients and particularly on consent to treatment. (para. 39)

From its inception, the MHAC has expressed concerns about the narrowness of its remit. The first Biennial Report drew attention to those groups, whose civil rights may be compromised, but who do not fall under the purview of the MHAC. The majority of people with mental handicap (now termed learning disability), following the introduction of the concept of mental impairment, no longer come within the provisions of the Mental Health Act, unless there is associated "abnormally aggressive or seriously irresponsible conduct." Even when patients with learning disability could be classified as mentally impaired, they may still be admitted to hospital as informal patients, if they are unable to make decisions for themselves (see below). Sometimes, the Commissioners come across units catering for patients with learning disability, where standards of care may be poor, and yet they may not have authority to intervene if the unit in question does not cater for detained patients. They may only become aware of such examples by chance, as was reported in the Ninth Biennial Report (2001).

> Patients resident on the men's villa (none of whom were detained under the Act) were housed on a locked ward in appalling conditions. A strong smell of urine pervaded the ward, and patients had little or no available activities or access to fresh air. The Commissioner recorded that she was shocked at the conditions and the aura of low expectations on the unit. It was even more disturbing that, as there were no detained patients on the ward, these conditions had come to the Commission's attention by chance.

Another group, which falls outside the MHAC's remit, comprises certain categories of children. The route by which a young person is detained in hospital can be somewhat arbitrary. Those admitted via the Children Act or directly by parents do not have access to the same rigorous framework for protection provided by the Mental Health Act, which includes the right to a second opinion, access to hospital managers' reviews and tribunal hearings, MHAC visits and entitlement to Section 117 aftercare.

The MHAC has also highlighted the position of mentally disordered offenders in prison. Even when they have been assessed as needing transfer for treatment in hospital, they are often left waiting for a place in prison. The MHAC does not have the power to monitor what is happening to them. They may remain languishing in prison, only to be transferred close to their release date, thereby reinforcing their feelings of grievance and their view of the transfer to hospital as a further 'punishment without end' (Eighth Biennial Report, p.95).

An overriding concern throughout the existence of the MHAC has been the position of incapacitated patients, who are compliant and have been admitted informally but who would be prevented from leaving hospital should they attempt to do so. The Third Biennial Report (1987-89) describes the position as follows:

> In one hospital, visiting Commissioners found there were 12 locked wards, but only a few had patients formally detained under the Mental Health Act. The problem has been intensified by the closure of hospitals and the movement of such patients into the private and voluntary sectors. ... Not infrequently Commissioners observe that professionals and staff do not always recognise the extent to which some of their patients are being deprived of their liberty. ... Just as frequently there is such recognition and extreme concern is often expressed to Commissioners about the lack of a clear legal and practice framework within which to take decisions about this group of patients.

The MHAC repeatedly urged the Secretary of State to exercise his/her power under Section 121(4) of the Act and extend the remit of the Commission to enable it to keep under review the care and treatment of de facto detained patients. The gap in the law relating to the position of these patients was later exposed in the Bournewood case.[12] This case put further pressure on the government to introduce legislative change.

The fact that the MHAC's remit only relates to those detained or liable to be detained in hospital has meant that it only has a limited role in relation to community care. It does enquire about the availability of mental health practitioners (ASWs and Section 12 doctors) to carry out assessments of people in the community who are being considered for compulsory admission. It will also look at the availability of aftercare services which will facilitate the discharge of patients. However, it has no power to keep the use of Guardianship or Supervised Discharge under review, except, in the latter case, during the application process which takes place while the patient is still subject to detention in hospital.

The remit of the Mental Health Commission in Scotland extended further than its sister body in that its duty covers all mentally disordered persons, incapable of adequately protecting themselves or their interests, whether they are in hospital, residential care homes or in their own homes. The Scottish Commission must be notified of all episodes of compulsory detention and community care orders. Unlike the MHAC, it may also recommend to the Secretary of State the discharge of patients from liability to detention or community care orders.

---

12 R v Bournewood Community and Mental Health Trust ext parte L [1998] 3 AER.

Visits to Hospitals

The primary way in which the MHAC carries out its task of protecting the interests of detained patients is by visiting and interviewing them in hospitals. The purpose of the visits is not to undertake detailed investigations, but to deal with issues raised by detained patients, to review how the Act is working and to observe how the interests of detained patients are being looked after.

In the early years, the aim was to ensure that each hospital or home was visited at least once a year. (Multi-disciplinary teams visited between 500 and 700 hospitals/ mental nursing homes each year.) Special Hospitals (now called High Secure Hospitals) were visited more frequently so that each high secure patient would have the opportunity of meeting with a Commissioner once a year. Meetings also took place with Social Service Departments to keep under review the co-ordination between hospital and community services of all aspects of a patient's detention from the initial assessment to the termination of aftercare.

This method of visiting meant that only a small proportion of detained patients were seen by a Commissioner, given that the duration of stay in hospital is only about 21 days and most patients were in and out between MHAC visits. In 1995, it was decided to restructure the MHAC in order to increase the quality and quantity of contact time between members of the MHAC and patients.

The number of commissioners was increased from 90 to up to 170 drawn, as before, from the range of disciplines in mental health and, on average, committing two or three days a month to Commission activity. Two types of Commissioner were appointed – full and visiting member. The main function of the latter was to meet with patients. Full visits were reduced to one every two years and more frequent (twice-yearly) Patient Focused Visits were introduced where the emphasis was placed on meeting detained patients rather than reviewing the range of services and facilities provided by the hospital.

The MHAC Secretariat has over 30 staff, providing administrative support to the visiting teams, and managing the Second Opinion Appointed Doctor referrals and other MHAC activities, such as the complaints and policy functions of the Commission.

According to the Ninth Biennial Report (2001, p.100), Commissioners made 22,593 direct patient contacts over the two year reporting period (about the same frequency of contact as the Lunacy Commissioners – see above). It also undertakes over 8,000 second opinions in each year.

Whatever the pattern of visiting, it has not been possible to measure the improvements in the care and treatment of detained patients which might have flowed directly from the MHAC visits. Admitting as much in his Chairman's Introduction to the Third Biennial Report, Louis Blom-Cooper maintained, however, that it was possible, by way of examples, to illustrate substantial changes which have been made to service provision. The Third Biennial Report proceeds to describe the case of one ward at Fulbourne Hospital, where, during 1986-88, the MHAC identified a series of problems concerning:

- The heterogeneous mix of patients.
- The poor state of the ward; in particular the inadequate number of tables and chairs for patients to sit at, the lack of separate washing and toilet facilities for women, dirty walls, torn upholstery, insufficient cutlery, an unsafe seclusion room and the absence of patient activities.
- The death of one patient from self-inflicted cerebral damage and another from suffocation on his own vomit. A further patient died unexpectedly and there were two other serious incidents.
- The lack of sufficient trained nursing staff and morale so low that on one visit, the ward nursing team handed Commissioners a memorandum saying "We can hardly maintain an adequate level of care … cannot progress further with rehabilitation." Detained patients also begged visiting Commissioners to seek improvements.

The MHAC made extra visits to the hospital (including one unannounced), met with senior managers of the hospital and the health authority and called for the allocation of further resources to ensure that the duty of care to detained patients was fulfilled. As a direct result of these activities, the Authority committed itself to a substantial increase in revenue expenditure, which made it possible for the hospital management immediately to make both structural and staffing improvements.

Many similar examples of the MHAC instigating significant improvements after identifying very poor standards can be found in later Biennial Reports. They found particularly poor conditions in hospitals due for closure at some point in the future, but which continued to house detained patients in appalling conditions. In the Fourth Biennial Report, a visit to Rainhill Hospital revealed one ward for 31 long stay mentally ill patients in a dismal state of deterioration with damp walls, broken chairs and only two baths positioned at the entrance to the ward, with a torn curtain and broken curtain rail, which deprived patients of any privacy. Another ward on the second floor, approached by a cement spiral staircase which appeared to have been used as a lavatory, was in equally bad condition. Strong representation from the MHAC, alongside other agencies, led to the wards being closed within a week and in a follow-up visit one month later the MHAC found that many patients had been transferred to new community facilities and those remaining were in greatly improved conditions.

Commissioners would also pursue issues raised from the meetings held in private with detained patients. While many of these issues might be regarded as trivial matters regarding everyday life on the ward, they could make a significant difference to the individual's period in hospital.

While the MHAC can point to many instances where conditions were improved both for the individual and the provider unit, standards in general have remained variable. There are also examples where, despite regular visiting, the MHAC has failed to expose sub-standard care. The Report of the Committee of Inquiry into Complaints about Ashworth Hospital in 1992 came to a series of disturbing conclusions about the regime and painted a picture "of life in a brutalising, stagnant, closed institution" (Fifth Biennial Report, p.23). Following this report, the MHAC accepted that it should have done more to uncover the impoverishment of patient care in the institution. It was evident that patients came to see the Commissioners as just part of the establishment of the hospital and that they were perceived as powerless in relation to the resolution of individual complaints made by high secure patients. However, there are real difficulties in any outside visitorial body 'getting under the skin of a total institution' and obtaining verifiable information. A similar problem arose in a second major inquiry at Ashworth Hospital, the Fallon Inquiry, which investigated the lax supervision in the Personality Disorder Unit. Here the MHAC escaped criticism, as the nefarious activities (misuse of drugs and alcohol, financial irregularities, possible paedophile activity and the availability of pornographic material) were so well hidden from view.

Throughout its existence, the MHAC has drawn attention to the issue of race and mental health. The first public conference which the MHAC held in 1987, attended by 300 participants, was on the theme "Better Mental Health Care for Ethnic Communities". In the Second Biennial Report, published later in the same year, the MHAC selected black and ethnic minority issues as one of its priority areas and made the following recommendations:

i.   Health and social services should formulate a policy and make adequate provision to meet the different needs of mentally disordered people from black and ethnic minority groups;

ii. Health and social services should designate a senior member of staff to take a special responsibility for this area;

iii. Health and social services with substantial populations whose first languages are other than English should employ qualified staff who speak these languages and, as an interim measure, establish good interpretation services;

iv. Health and social services should gather information on the number of patients from black and ethnic minority communities;

v.   The Secretary of State should seek nominations of individuals with appropriate experience and qualifications from black and minority groups for membership of the Commission.

The MHAC endorsed the approach of a few hospitals (Bradford, Rochdale, Tameside and Oldham) that were attempting to help patients from black and ethnic minority communities maintain familiar patterns of daily living and keep in touch with their own communities. However, the majority of hospitals expected all patients to conform to the hospital's routines and customs, perpetuating among members of ethnic communities a feeling of alienation and leading to strongly critical attitudes towards the mental health service as a whole (Second Biennial Report, p.51).

The response of mental health services to the repeated exhortations of the MHAC in successive Biennial Reports has been slow, prompting the Commission to comment 10 years later in the Seventh Biennial Report (1997):

Provision for patients from ethnic minority communities often remains basic, insensitive and piecemeal, leading to patients feeling alienated and isolated. It is dispiriting that the serious issues of inappropriate care and treatment of patients from black and ethnic communities, which were raised in previous Biennial Reports, continue to cause concern and be noted in reports of Commission Visits. (p.171)

The importance of making mental health services more responsive to the needs of black ethnic groups is reinforced by the fact that they are greatly over-represented among detained patients. Figures collected by the MHAC itself revealed that the number of patients detained from black ethnic groups was five or six times the proportion of such groups in the population. The use for Asian groups was roughly in line with the expected number, which also raises questions of whether their problems are being hidden.

The MHAC decided to take a more proactive stance to promote change and, in 1999, undertook a National Visit, in which 117 units were visited on the same day, to build up a nationwide picture of current policies and practice with particular reference to three target areas, ethnic monitoring, the use of interpreters and racial harassment.

The MHAC's drive to highlight race equality issues culminated in a national census of the ethnicity of people using in-patient mental health services. It was carried out in collaboration with the Healthcare Commission and the National Institute for Mental Health in England and took place on 31 March 2005.[13] It covered almost 34,000 mental health inpatients, using services provided by 102 NHS Trusts and 110 independent providers in England and Wales. Among the key findings was that rates of admission into hospital were three or more times higher for black and white-black mixed groups compared with the average. Rates of admission were particularly high in the 'Other Black' category, largely comprising young black people born in the UK. From among this hospital population, black groups were up to 44 per cent more likely to be detained under the Mental Health Act. Black Caribbean and Black African groups were almost twice as likely as other ethnic groups to be referred through the criminal justice system. There were also higher rates of the use of restraint (29 per cent higher than average for Black Caribbean men) and seclusion (50 per cent higher for men from Black and Indian ethnic groups).

Another area, in which the MHAC has striven to make improvements but has hit a brick wall, is the delays in transfers from high secure hospitals to a less secure environment. Not only do these excessive delays constitute an inappropriate and wasteful use of expensive high secure places, but it is de-motivating for the patient and undermines one of the principles of the Code of Practice that patients should be "given any necessary treatment or care in the least controlled and segregated facilities compatible with ensuring their own health or safety or the safety of other people" (para. 1.1). In the late 1980s, the MHAC conducted studies at Rampton and Moss Side Hospitals of patients whose transfer had been delayed for over two and three years. The efforts of the MHAC to expedite transfers were thwarted firstly because of protracted Home Office consideration of the case and then because of inability or unwillingness of consultants in local hospitals to offer a bed. In the Ninth Biennial Report, the MHAC were still commenting on the lack of progress, drawing attention

---

13 Commission for Healthcare Audit and Inspection (2005) *Count me in*. Results of a national census of inpatients in mental health hospitals and facilities in England and Wales.

to the fact that there were, in April 2001, 349 patients in the transfer/discharge system within the High Security Hospitals, 27 per cent of the total patient population in the three hospitals. The MHAC also pointed out that this figure does not take account of the numbers who are not yet on the list because there is no realistic hope of finding them alternative accommodation.

The Collection of Data

The Lunacy Commission and the Board of Control received returns from each institution about every detention and other details about various interventions, such as the use of restraint, seclusion and sedation. Following in these footsteps, the MHAC identified "more effective collection of data for reviewing the working of the Act" as one of its priorities in the First Biennial Report. However, the MHAC has not had the tools in terms of staffing, technical know-how or computer equipment to make this possible.

While in Scotland the Mental Welfare Commission receives notification of all compulsory admissions, in England the statistical branch of the Department of Health has taken on the role of receiving and analysing data on the operation of the Act. The DoH data has serious limitations. Apart from gender, information is not linked to other patient characteristics, such as ethnicity, age and socio-economic circumstances. From the mid 1990s, the MHAC attempted to supplement the DoH data with the collection of some additional information concerning such matters as the ethnicity of patients who had been subject to the Act, the use of seclusion and tribunal and managers' hearings. There was still an obvious need for more systematic research. In its Seventh Biennial Report (1997), the MHAC called for research to examine some of the factors which underlie statistical trends in the use of the Act. As part of the review of the 1983 Act, the DoH did respond by commissioning an extensive series of research reports (Shaping the New Mental Health Act). The SSI also published a Report of the ASW role in compulsory admissions (Detained). Incredibly, the MHAC failed to make any reference to these studies in its Ninth Biennial Report, even on the study evaluating the quantitative and qualitative data accumulated by the Mental Health Act Commission itself (Shaw, Middleton et al., see next chapter). This is despite the fact that it was advocating, at the time, that its successor body should take on responsibility for information collection.

As far as its own activities are concerned, the MHAC is able to supply data on its input (i.e. finance and staffing), output (the number and type of visits, second opinions and complaints). However, it has produced little statistical data on the outcomes, particularly in relation to quantifying the nature of the observations it has made on visits, the recommendations made and whether services have responded. This gap has only partly been filled by Shaw and Middleton's study. The brief which the DoH gave the researchers was restricted to evaluating the information the MHAC holds, both qualitative, in the shape of its visit reports, and quantitative, the second opinion data. Unfortunately, it did not include any fieldwork research, and missed an opportunity to evaluate the impact the MHAC has had on service provision.

In more recent years, the MHAC has begun to collect data in a more systematic way. It undertook two National Visits. Over 100 hospitals were visited in one day with the aim of obtaining a national picture of issues of central importance to the care and treatment of detained patients. The matters investigated in the first National Visit in 1996 were the number, qualifications and deployment of staff, policies and procedures concerning leave for detained patients and the safety and privacy of women patients. An example of one of the observations which Commissioners made during this Visit was that there was no nurse interacting with patients on a quarter of the wards visited and where there was interaction, staff were mainly engaged in one-to-one observations with little therapeutic input. The Second National Visit (1999), as has been mentioned, examined the care and treatment of detained patients from black and ethnic minority communities.

In 1998, the MHAC introduced a procedure, Matters Requiring Particular Attention (MRPA) whereby a small number of selected items were monitored on every visit with the intention of reporting the findings in the Biennial Report. During the reporting period covered by the Ninth Biennial Report, the MRPA topics were: statutory information given to patients, contact with the Responsible Medical Officer, the operation of a 'named' nurse system and ECT facilities. It was reported that, in almost a quarter of units visited, staff were unable to identify when and by whom individual patients' rights were explained and that a small but sizeable proportion of facilities did not have leaflets explaining the rights of patients who are detained under Section 2 or 3. No findings relating to the level of contact with the Responsible Medical Officer or whether patients were allocated a 'named' nurse or equivalent were published and, while some findings on the ECT survey were reported, a promise to "publish a fuller picture of policy and practice relating to ECT administration" (Ninth Biennial Report, p.31) was not fulfilled.

The MHAC extended the system of collecting standardised information by introducing a new visiting format. Commissioners were expected to administer a series of Commission Visiting Questionnaires in an attempt to provide a better "evidential base" of MHAC visits. There is a strong argument for greater standardisation in the collection of information from visits. Shaw and Middleton in their evaluation of MHAC data found inconsistencies and differences of approach between visiting teams and recommended a more strongly centralised approach to defining the conduct of visits. More uniform procedures should enable current standards to be ascertained and realistic targets to be set to improve practice. There is also a need for good record keeping where matters of liberty are concerned. However, there is a limit to the amount of data which can be collected in this way. It was noted above how the statistical information collected by the Lunacy Commission increased in bulk and importance, but they were unable to make other than the "most plain and obvious deductions." Similarly, the MHAC has not got a good track record in making good use of the information it collects. There are also issues and concerns relating to the circumstances of individual patients and particular units which can only be ascertained by Commissioners using their professional expertise. Some Commissioners felt alienated by what they saw as the increasing bureaucratisation of the MHAC (see discussion below). The introduction of checklists as the main means of collecting data on visits resulted in disaffection among some Commissioners, who did not feel that ticking boxes on forms is making full use of their professional skills (personal communications).

The Final Years of the Mental Health Act Commission

The MHAC has been described as 'a toothless watchdog'. Indeed, its capacity to be a major driving force for change in mental health services has been limited by its weak remit, uncertain status and inadequate funding. However its influence has exceeded its powers because of the knowledge and expertise of its membership. One of the strengths of the MHAC has been its ability to recruit members of high calibre from diverse professional backgrounds. In March 2001, its membership was recorded as consisting of nearly half from a nursing or social work background, 15 per cent lawyers, 11 per cent consultant psychiatrists or GPs and 26 per cent from other disciplines such as psychology, pharmacy or mental health administration or from non-professional backgrounds. A number of Commissioners are or have been service users or carers. Just under half are female and over 20 per cent are from black and minority ethnic groups (Ninth Biennial Report, p.98).

Rules limiting the tenure of public appointments have meant that there is a regular turnover of members. Unlike the Lunacy Commission, where Lord Ashley was Chairman for 40 years and other members stayed in post until their dotage, the MHAC has had a series of Chairmen. The first was Lord Colville of Culross (1983-87), a former Home Office Minister, who was succeeded in turn by Louis Blom-Cooper QC (1987-94), a barrister, Dame Ruth Runciman (1994-98), former Chairman of the Prison Reform Trust and having served on advisory bodies on the misuse of drugs, Gordon Lakes CB MC (acting 1998-99), ex-Deputy Director-General of the Prison Service, and Margaret Clayton (1999-2002), who was a permanent under-secretary at the Home Office. The current incumbent is Professor Lord Kamlesh Patel OBE, Head of the Centre for Ethnicity & Health and Institute for Philosophy, Diversity and Mental Health. He was also National Director of the Department of Health black and minority ethnic mental health programme and was appointed to the House of Lords in 2006. Some continuity was provided by William Bingley, who was chief executive throughout the 1990s. He had a mental health law background, having been legal officer for MIND and also having been seconded to the Department of Health to draft the first edition of the Code of Practice. His leadership enhanced the reputation of the MHAC both within the organisation and in the mental health services as a whole.

Paul Hampshire was appointed Chief Executive in 2000, but was only in post for two years, resigning suddenly with an £80,000 pay off. In his pen picture posted on the MHAC website at the time of his appointment, he confessed that he had no knowledge or experience in mental health, his background being in local government and health authority finance and audit. He was intent on introducing a more systematic approach to visiting. A more bureaucratic approach was adopted, encouraging 'self regulation and self assessment processes' among provider units, while the MHAC would take on a 'validating', 'quality re-assurance role'. In defence of this new approach, the MHAC argued that

We do not share the view that good management systems are a bureaucratic end in themselves. We believe that good systems are major cogs to connect the engine of policy to the wheels of practice so that detained patients actually receive the service intended by the legislation and related guidance. (Ninth Biennial Report, p.109)

On the other hand, there was a view that one of the original purposes of the MHAC to be "a forum for inter-professional discussion of issues concerning the law and ethics on the treatment of detained patients" (White Paper, 1981, quoted above) was being undermined. The Legal and Ethical Special Interest Group was abandoned. The once highly successful programme of training, which gave managers and practitioners the opportunity to explore with Commissioners how any problems in implementing the Code of Practice might be overcome in particular localities, ground to a halt. The MHAC Guidance Notes, which give advice on matters not included in the Code of Practice, were not kept up to date. The MHAC website, set up in 2000 and including at that time a summary of the significant mental health case laws, was allowed to stagnate.

In a stinging critique of the Ninth Biennial Report, Eldergill comments:

... the Commission has generated 75 recommendations that require services to devise at least 98 staff intensive, often bureaucratic steps, many of which have nothing to do with the 1983 Act ... Assuming for a moment that this is a proper function for a Mental Health Act Commission, does this help professionals to provide better mental health services? The disadvantages are obvious: too many quality-assurance commissions, too much top-down guidance, too many codes of practice, confusion on the ground about what to prioritise, a feeling amongst staff that they are drowning in policies and procedures, the impossibility of meeting all targets, demoralisation, and so on.

These faults were compounded by the MHAC's Chief Executive's follow-up letter to the Biennial Report of 21 June 2002 sent to local mental health service managers. The letter referred to "more positive management control arrangements" advocated in the MHAC's Ninth Biennial Report and the recommendation that "local self-assessment or clinical audit style review procedures be developed as an integral part of your quality assurance programme regarding the use of the Act and Code of Practice." It was accompanied by a "standardised summary report of self-assessment recommendations for mental health providers" – i.e. a checklist which had 14 areas for assessment and five assessment criteria with a possible red, amber, green response giving a total of 210 boxes. There was another checklist for mental health commissioners. Eldergill (op cit) refers to "a general weariness about the endless raft of guidance and recommendations and professionals opening their post may be seen 'binning' what they regard as the NHS equivalent of the innovations catalogue inserted in daily newspapers."

In fact, according to the Tenth Biennial Report,[14] only about one quarter (72) of all detaining hospitals in England and Wales bothered to return the self-assessment schedules. The validity of such self-assessment reports must also be open to doubt.

---

14 The Mental Health Act Commission (2003) *Tenth Biennial Report 2001-2003. Placed amongst strangers. Twenty years of the Mental Health Act 1983 and future prospects for compulsion*, London: TSO.

For example, Commissioners in their own survey of seclusion facilities, using the Commission visiting questionnaire, found that compliance with Code of Practice standards with regard to such matters as privacy, safety, and the adequacy of furnishings, heating, lighting and ventilation to be poor (with well over a 50 per cent failure rate). Only a small minority of the units, who assessed themselves, recorded that the availability and compliance with written policies on seclusion to be 'in the red' or even 'amber'.

Following the appointment of Christopher Heginbotham as Chief Executive in 2003, the MHAC shifted its emphasis back towards listening to the voice of the detained patient. Christopher Heginbotham was director of MIND in the 1980s and then held a number of chief executive positions in the NHS. The number of Commissioners was reduced to about 120 part-time members. Two types of Commissioner were appointed; a Local Commissioner, who visits detained patients, examines statutory records, takes up immediate issues on behalf of the patient and identifies priorities, which require follow-up action concerning the ward environment and culture or legal issues; and an Area Commissioner, who co-ordinates the work of the Commission within a strategic health authority or Welsh region, developing relationships with providers, social services, user groups and other agencies and writes annual reports, which are presented to the Boards of providers. Commissioners were required, once again, to be credible, autonomous representatives of the Mental Health Act Commission.

A new visiting regime was introduced, which moved away from formal one-off visits towards a system whereby a Commissioner, working on their own, would carry out short notice or unannounced visits to meet with patients and check statutory documents. The target was to:

- visit every unit with detained patients at least once per annum;
- visit every ward with detained patients at least once every 18 months;
- meet and interview 20 per cent of all detained patients in every year.

The purpose of the visits is to observe the conditions in which patients are detained, to ensure the lawfulness of detention and to offer guidance on the implementation of the Act and Code of Practice. Commission visiting questionnaires are not used in a routine way, buts as a tool to monitor compliance with specific areas of the Act, as and when relevant. Feedback is given on the day of the visit with the intention of resolving issues at ward level, as far as possible. There is no formal report after each visit, but information is collated for inclusion in an annual report provided for each NHS Trust and independent hospital.

The Tenth Biennial Report of the Commission matched this change in direction. The focus of the Report was not just to ensure that the Mental Health Act and Code of Practice procedures are carried out correctly, but that their underlying purpose, the protection of the human rights of patients, is fulfilled in spirit as well as in form, and that the voice of the individual service user is heard. This is reflected in the title, "Placed Amongst Strangers", which was given to the Report. This was the expression used by John Perceval[15] in an account of his experience of detention in the 1830s, in which he referred to the fact that not only was he deprived of his liberty and "placed amongst strangers, without introduction, explanation or exhortation" but that also "on every occasion, in every dispute, in every argument, the assumed premise immediately acted upon was that I was to yield, my desires were to be set aside, my few remaining privileges to be infringed upon for the convenience of others." The Tenth Biennial Report draws out the similarities between the complaints of John Perceval 160 years ago (the lack of information about his circumstances and reasons for detention, the imposition of restrictions beyond that which was necessary and the lack of choice about his care or treatment) and those of present day detained patients. The inference, the MHAC point out, is that the deprivation of liberty and/or the use of compulsion for reasons of mental disorder, usually through no fault of the person concerned, is such a serious interference with human rights that there will always be a need for a visitorial body charged specifically with monitoring the application of powers and discharge of duties covered by mental health legislation.

---

15 John Perceval was the son of Prime Minister, Spencer Perceval, who was assassinated in 1812. He was one of the founder members of the Alleged Lunatic's Friend Society. See Mental Health Act Commission (2003) Tenth Biennial Report; pp.22 and 23.

Chapter 3

Exploring Visiting Activities of the Commission

Ian Shaw, Hugh Middleton and Martin Chamberlain

The Remit and Visiting Policy of the Commission

The Mental Health Act Commission (MHAC) undertakes visits to the three Special Hospitals (Ashworth, Rampton and Broadmoor), Trusts, Social Service Departments and Mental Nursing Homes to fulfil its duties under Section 120 of the 1983 Mental Health Act in respect to:

- keeping under review the exercise of the powers and duties contained in the Act which relate to detained patients and to patients liable to be detained;
- visiting and interviewing in private patients detained under the Act in hospital and nursing homes.

The Commission is a visitorial body and not an inspectorate. Consequently, the Code of Practice is the Commission's source of 'quality control' when undertaking its visiting duties.

The Commission operates on a two year visiting cycle from 1 April to 31 March, the conclusion of which coincides with the publication of a Biennial Report.

From 1990 the Commission centralised the management of its visiting activities in Nottingham. Consequently visiting Commissioners were attached to one of seven regional areas (CVTs 1 to 7) or one of the three High Security Hospitals. Each CVT area has its day-to-day visiting arrangements co-ordinated by a CVT Convenor, supported by the MHAC Administration staff based in Nottingham. Overall responsibility for the visit policy and programme lies with the Commissions Policy Committee.

Different types of visits are undertaken. Briefly these are:

- Full or Joint (when Social Services are included) Visits – where the focus is on the range of services offered by the Trust and Social Service Departments. During these visits Commissioners meet with a wide range of Trust and/or Social Service Managers and Regional Purchasing Authority representatives. Separate visits can also be undertaken to Social Service Departments. One Full or Joint Visit is undertaken in a two-year visiting cycle. When Social Service Departments are separately visited, one visit to each is undertaken during the two-year period.

- Patient Focused – where the focus is upon meeting detained patients and reviewing their detention documents. A minimum of three Patient Focused Visits are undertaken in a two-year visiting cycle.
- Unannounced Visits – currently, unannounced visits count for 10 per cent of all visits as a matter of MHAC policy. These can also be undertaken in response to a particular concern (i.e. continuing concerns with the physical environment on wards).
- Targeted Visits – these are either undertaken as part of an MHAC review of a particular issue (i.e. use of Seclusion) or like Unannounced Visits in response to a specific concern.
- Short Notice and Out of Hours (weekend/night) Visits – these are also undertaken if deemed necessary. It is possible to have a Targeted Unannounced or Short Notice Out of Hours Visit.

On visits, Commissioners are guided by the Commission's Visiting Policy. This provides advice and aide-memoirs on specific areas of interest relevant to the different types of visit, the Mental Health Act and Code of Practice. It also includes guidance upon how the different types of visit should be focused and organised, and the format in which reports should be produced. Page three of the Commission's Visiting Policy details the essential purpose of the Commission's Visits. These are:

Hospitals and Mental Nursing Homes

Visits by members of the Commission to hospitals and mental nursing homes have, broadly speaking, a fourfold purpose:

1. to meet with detained patients in private , particularly those who have asked to meet members of the Commission. Meetings may be with individual patients or with groups of patients, including Patients' Councils;
2. to observe the conditions in which patients are detained;
3. to see how the provisions of the Mental Health Act 1983 and the Code of Practice are being applied;
4. to offer advice and guidance on the implementation of the Act. The highest priority should be given to meeting detained patients and to checking the detention documents.

Social Service Departments

The purpose of meeting representatives of Social Service Departments is to encourage a co-ordinated approach to the operation of the Act and, in particular, to keep under review:

1. the Social Service Departments' response to the Act and the Code of Practice;

2. the process of assessment, compulsory admission and detention under the Act, including the availability of ASWs, communication with GPs, hospitals, Section 12 Doctors and the emergency services;
3. the planning and delivery of appropriate residential places, alternatives to detention and aftercare procedures and facilities;
4. the extent to which hospital and community services are able to integrate all aspects of a patient's detention from the initial assessment to the termination of aftercare.

Purchasers

The purpose of meeting representatives of the relevant purchasing authorities is to ensure that the contractual arrangements meet the needs of the detained patients, that the services being delivered meet the contractual requirements, and to help and encourage the purchasers to engage in the routine monitoring of service delivery. Meetings with both purchasers and providers should enable the Commission to gain a better insight into the quality and pattern of mental health services.

The Commission Policy: including its requirement to give highest priority to meeting detained patients and checking detention documentation, the different types of visit that are undertaken, information received prior to the undertaking of a visit and the specific type of Trust, or ward, to be visited (for example Learning Disability) all effect the content of the subsequent visit report forwarded to a Trust upon the completion of a visit. This is acknowledged in Part C, page C 9 of the Commissions Policy & Procedures Document concerning the Commission's checklist of topics that may be considered during a visit. It is stressed here, however, that all areas of interest should be considered at some time in the two-year visiting cycle.

The Visiting Process

Organisation and Initial Data Requested

Unless a visit is to be unannounced, the MHAC inform the Trust, Mental Nursing Home or Social Service Department of the intended date on which the visit will take place. Information on the number of detained patients by ward, sex, ethnicity and the current Section they are detained under is requested, as is information concerning the availability of copies of, and training in, the Code of Practice and Mental Health Act on wards. An annual statistical return concerning the Trust's use of the Act (know as Hospital Profile Statistics) can also be requested, depending upon the length of time since the last visit undertaken by the Commission. Once received, the above, along with copies of the last Commission report, are forwarded to visiting Commissioners for their information. Any other pertinent information, such as patient deaths since the last visit, or correspondence received from patients, staff or other interested parties such as voluntary organisations, is also forwarded to visiting Commissioners.

Meetings and Data Collected

Visits start and end with meetings with Trust or Nursing Home representatives. On Unannounced, Patient Focused, Targeted, or Out of Hours Visits this may primarily be with a Mental Health Act Administrator or other named contact. On Full Visits, where initial discussion regarding service developments is required, Senior Trust Managers, representatives from the Police and Ambulance Services, alongside Voluntary Organisations and other interested parties such as patient groups or GP collectives, can be present at these meetings; or met at some point during the visit. On visits to, or which include, Social Service Departments, meetings with Approved Social Workers and senior Social Service staff occur. Representatives from Purchasing Authorities are also invited to meet Commissioners.

During visits, Commissioners observe the condition of facilities provided for detained patients, hold private meetings with detained patients at their request and scrutinise legal documentation. Issues concerning patients' documentation are discussed with the most senior ward nurse on duty at the time of the visit, while patients who hold a private meeting with Commissioners receive a letter outlining the content of their discussion with the Commissioner and any further action agreed. A copy of this is given to ward staff if the patient wishes it. Issues requiring urgent attention – such as where a patient may be illegally detained due to errors in their documentation – are followed up and a specific time limit for a response may be requested.

Commissioners collect information concerning their contact with patients (Section detained under, age, sex, ethnicity and issue raised) and more recently have started collecting data concerning what are called 'Matters Requiring Particular Attention'. This has been collected on every Patient Focused Visit since 1997, though difficulties with this process mean data is only available from 1998. The topics are – forms 38 (Consent to Treatment), seclusion, the physical examination of patients, women's care and ethnic monitoring. For 1999/2000 the topics selected are: statutory information given to patients; contact with the Responsible Medical Officer; the operation of a 'named' nurse or equivalent system; and ECT facilities.

The meeting held at the end of a visit concerns the Commission's findings. It is a matter of policy to highlight good as well as poor practice both in this meeting and in the subsequent visit report.

Distribution of the Visit Report

Shortly after a visit has finished the Commissioners involved discuss the content of the report. A drafting process then begins which involves the Commission's administration staff. Once completed a copy is forwarded to the relevant Mental Nursing Home, Trust and/or Social Service Department. Copies are also sent to the relevant Purchasing Authority. The report will contain areas of general and specific concern and possibly issues where specific responses within a time limit are requested.

When the response to the report is received, copies are immediately sent to the visiting Commissioners by the administration staff in Nottingham. If this is unsatisfactory in some respects, subsequent correspondence or a further visit may occur. Similarly the lack of a response within a certain timeframe may result in a further visit being undertaken in the near future if it is felt necessary.

The current practice of the Commission is for each CVT Convenor to produce half-yearly reports concerning the general conditions under which patients are detained and the implementation of the Mental Health Act and Code of Practice in their respective CVT area. These are forwarded to the Commission's Policy Co-ordinator and used to inform the organisation of the Commission's Visiting Programme and identify trends to be included in Biennial Reports.

Visit reports and the replies they generate, along with all correspondence concerning each Special Hospital, Trust, Mental Nursing Home or Social Service Department received by the Commission's administration staff are stored in the Commission's offices. Each has its own distinct file stored by the CVT area in which it is visited. The Special Hospitals have their own distinct visiting arrangements and so are filed separately.

The Commission's administration staff manage these files and the correspondence contained within them. Commission reports and responses to them vary in size; on average they are each around five pages in length.

The Commission's Review of its Visit Operations

As detailed in Chapter 3 of its Eighth Biennial Report, the Commission has reviewed its visiting policy. This review has led to a reduction in the number of Patient Focused Visits from three to two, along with the refocusing of the distinction between Full and Patient Focused Visits and the purpose of visits to Social Service Departments.

In addition the Commission's Policy Co-ordinator has advised each CVT Convenor of changes concerning the format of reports forwarded to him and the Commission is currently undertaking a review of its information technology systems.

From its visits, the MHAC collects a large amount of data concerning its implementation of the Act and Code of Practice. As already noted it collects information via its Hospital Profile Statistics, contact with detained patients and the 'Matters Requiring Particular Attention' in addition to the data held in visit reports and their replies.

As this data is systematically collected and discussed in the MHAC Biennial Reports and that further information pertaining to contact with detained patients held in the Commission's files is of a confidential nature, it was felt necessary to specifically focus the analysis upon the data in the Commission's visit reports and the Trust's replies.

As already noted, currently each CVT Convenor produces a half-yearly report concerning the general trends within his or her CVT area, as the MHAC does not have the resources to systematically analyse the data held in its reports and replies. The data in the Commission's Biennial Report concerning its visiting programme is then the distillation of its visiting experience during a particular period and it was felt that a systematic analysis of this would enable comment to be made upon the current role of the Commission and its management of this data.

The Commission holds a large amount of data in its visit reports and Trust replies and, as this analysis is retrospective, it was felt necessary to focus on specific topics so that a degree of density within in the data could be obtained. Preliminary analysis revealed certain prevalent topics and we decided to concentrate specifically upon these in the first stage of analysis. In effect these topics arise from the scrutiny of detained patients' detention documentation, or from observing the general environment in which patients are or may be detained.

The Commission's Management of its Data

Overall the standard and accessibility of the Commission files relating to its visiting programme are excellent, though some are rather bulky. However, towards the end of the scanning of files for this project the Commission was undertaking a review of its documentation for forwarding to its off-site storage facility; during this time files are 'weeded', organised more accessibly and duplicate information removed.

This said the following discussion concerning the management of its visiting programme may be of interest to the Commission.

The current organisation of the Commission's database for the storage of files sent off-site consists of a set of box-files that contain slips of paper giving the relevant information when required. It is of concern that this system is not computerised and there do not appear to be back-up copies of these slips.

There are currently two instances of Trusts receiving insufficient visits. Of these two Trusts, the first one received a visit in March 1995 – which is just outside of the beginning of the sampled period – and then no other visit could be found in the Trust files until August 1997, subsequent visits being undertaken in September 1998 and March 1999.

Though this was of concern, the reasons surrounding the lack of visits for a second Trust are more so. This Trust was visited in 1994 and then was not visited until March 1998. In this case contact was made with the CVT Convenor responsible for the area in which this Trust is visited. This revealed that the Trust was 'forgotten' until, by chance, a fellow Commissioner inquired who visited its facilities. Though this type of occurrence is indeed rare, these two highlighted will be of interest to the Commission so it can ensure it fulfils the responsibilities it has under the Mental Health Act in regard to meeting detained patients and checking their detention documentation.

Finally, analysis of the Commission's visit reports has revealed that the data within them could be extracted and used as a monitoring tool to better effect than at present if further steps where made to ensure that they contained richer descriptions of issues than at present. From personal communication with the Commission's Policy Co-ordinator it was clear that a request had been made to CVT Convenors that their six-monthly summaries of visits undertaken in their CVT area are given via a pro-forma that asks for a comprehensive account of visit outcomes.

The majority of reports analysed gave a detailed account of the concerns expressed by Commissioners during visits. However, on occasion it is not possible to ascertain which areas of a Trust concerns relate to or the exact nature of the concerns in any more than general terms. This has limited the breath of the coding framework, particularly in regard to obtaining specific data on variation in practice within a Trust.

The following extract illustrates that Trusts can also on occasion feel a fuller description within reports would enable them to better address the concerns of the Commission.

> It would be helpful in the future if the Commission could provide specific details of when shortcomings are highlighted. The Trust would then be able to identify precisely who is responsible for a specific problem and have a more robust mandate with which to address it with them.

The following extracts relating to Section 132 of the Act illustrate the difference in the detail present in some Commission reports. Both extracts are taken from Full Visits to a number of wards within Trusts. Both do detail the essential nature of the Commissioner's concerns in regard to Section 132 of the Act, but the second extract provides a richer description of the variation in practice throughout the Trust's facilities.

> Section 132
> In some cases it was not clear whether the patient had understood their rights, even when they had been given information. Commissioners suggested that a formal record of understanding should be made by the informant primary nurse.

> Section 132
> Commissioners commended the form which is used to monitor the giving of rights information to patients within the Hospital. The form is well used on 'Smith' and 'Jones' Wards where the Commissioners found it a most useful document for monitoring rights information. On other wards its use appeared random. In 'Donald Ward' it appeared not to be in use at all. Commissioners requested that the use of this form is standardised throughout the Hospital.

Reports represent a summary of the scope of the Commission's visit and the issues of concern. They are qualitative documents written without the intention to subsequently systematically review them in comparison with each other and as such they are instances where their examination by somebody other than a Commissioner who undertook the visit would not reveal the full extent and nature of concerns expressed.

> Commissioners made reference to the number of Sections 5(2) which had been allowed to lapse.

If Commissioners where advised to complete reports more descriptively, a coding framework could be developed and used to monitor their content.

The implementation of such a system would not necessarily mean an increase in the strain on Commission resources. The Commission's administration staff were involved in the report drafting process and it would consequently have taken a relatively small period of time for them to transfer the data held in reports via a simple coding framework onto an electronic database. Such a database would prove invaluable in providing systematic data for the Commission's Biennial Report, monitoring visit activity, and trends in the use of the Mental Health Act and Code of Practice. Additionally such a database may allow the Commission to keep a record of where a current response to a Commission report does not discuss a particular issue raised in the report or where a reply has not been received by the Commission. The Commission is in the process of reviewing its current Information Technology requirements.

Topic Analysis

Figure 3.1 below shows the current frequency of instances of concern for coded topics as per the coding framework in Appendix One of this report. For topics with more than one issue to be accounted for (i.e. Consent to Treatment), the total number of reports that contain at least one instance of concern has been calculated.

TOPIC	95-97	97-99	CVT1	CVT2	CVT3	CVT4	CVT5	CVT6	CVT7	Total	Low	Medium	High
Consent (Forms 38 & 9)	207	332	82	81	81	44	105	63	83	539	159	191	189
Proportion (%)	38	62	15	15	15	8	19	12	15	100	29	35	35
Samples Proportion (%)			15	13	11	11	22	12	17	100	31	41	28
Section17	182	257	72	64	57	39	87	34	86	439	126	159	154
Proportion (%)	41	59	16	15	13	9	20	8	20	100	29	36	35
Samples Proportion (%)			15	13	11	11	22	12	17	100	31	41	28
Section 132	56	115	56	30	29	1	27	4	24	171	63	49	59
Proportion (%)	33	67	33	18	17	1	16	2	14	100	37	29	35
Samples Proportion (%)			15	13	11	11	22	12	17	100	31	41	28
Section 5(2)	80	81	35	19	26	13	30	16	22	161	51	53	57
Proportion (%)	50	50	22	12	16	8	19	10	14	100	32	33	35
Samples Proportion (%)			15	13	11	11	22	12	17	100	31	41	28
Ethnic Recording	17	104	44	37	3	11	15	3	8	121	53	32	36
Proportion (%)	14	86	36	31	2	9	12	2	7	100	44	26	30
Samples Proportion (%)			15	13	11	11	22	12	17	100	31	41	28
Physical Examination	16	83	43	32	4	3	8	7	2	99	53	19	27
Proportion (%)	16	84	43	32	4	3	8	7	2	100	54	19	27
Samples Proportion (%)			15	13	11	11	22	12	17	100	31	41	28
Section 136	45	47	12	12	17	5	3	16	27	92	21	37	34
Proportion (%)	49	51	13	13	18	5	3	17	29	100	23	40	37
Samples Proportion (%)			15	13	11	11	22	12	17	100	31	41	28
Section 12 Doctors	42	44	15	12	12	4	1	22	20	86	23	30	33
Proportion (%)	49	51	17	14	14	5	1	26	23	100	27	35	38
Samples Proportion (%)			15	13	11	11	22	12	17	100	31	41	28
AWOL	19	30	16	16	5	1	2	3	6	49	17	10	22
Proportion (%)	39	61	33	33	10	2	4	6	12	100	35	20	45
Samples Proportion (%)			15	13	11	11	22	12	17	100	31	41	28

Figure 3.1 Breakdown of Topics by Period, CVT and Mini Indicators

The number of instances of concern is shown by Period One and Period Two, by CVT area and then Mini score. The column labelled 'Total' immediately after the respective CVT area columns displays the total number of instances of concern in reports for each topic. Obviously this total is the same as the totals for Mini Scores & Periods.

The row immediately below each topic heading – 'Proportion (per cent)' – gives in percentage terms the relative frequency of the topic for each of the Period, CVT and Mini categories when calculated by the total number of instances of concern for that topic. For example, instances of concern in regard to Consent to Treatment (Forms 38 & 9) occur in total on 539 of the 789 visits. By CVTs 1 to 7 this breaks down as 82, 81, 81, 44, 105, 63 and 83 instances of concern respectively. When these totals are shown in proportion to the total number of instances, their values are 15 per cent, 15 per cent, 15 per cent, 8 per cent, 19 per cent, 12 per cent and 15 per cent respectively.

The row below 'Proportion (per cent)' – 'Sample Proportion (per cent)' – relates to the proportion in percentage terms of the number of Trusts in the sample by both CVT and Mini indicators respectively. So, for example, 31 per cent of the 94 Trusts sampled have a low Mini score, 41 per cent Medium Mini score and 28 per cent a High Mini score. This then is giving a baseline from which to at first compare a topic by CVT area, Mini and Period categories.

Though the sample is incomplete, it appears that the data as it stands is showing that instances of concern occur more frequently in Trusts with High Mini scores then those with Low and Medium Mini scores, with the notable exception of Ethnic Recording and the Physical Examination of Patients respectively. Here Low Mini scores seem to be over-represented. Discussion of this situation and that the Commission was able to shed some light on it is in the Commission's "Matters Requiring Particular Attention".

Though overall CVTs 1, 2 and 3 appear to have a higher proportion of instances of concern for topics in comparison to other CVTs, the majority of instances where there are differences relate to the CVT areas which require further data, in particular CVTs 4 and 6.

When all Topics are coded and required data retrieved from the Commission's off-site facility, the data will become clearer and more comprehensive. It is expected at this time that the topics most frequently reported as being of concern – currently Consent to Treatment, Section 17, the recording of Patient Rights and the use of Section 5(2) – will be subject to statistical tests using SPSS to gauge significance by CVT and Mini Indicators. Brief discussion of each topic follows.

Section 5(2) Doctors' Holding Powers

The Doctors' Holding enables the detention of an informal patient for up to 72 hours to allow consideration of an application under Section 2 or 3.

Code	95-97	97-99	CVT1	CVT2	CVT3	CVT4	CVT5	CVT6	CVT7	Low	Medium	High	Total
Section 5(4)	80	81	35	19	26	13	30	16	22	51	53	57	161
Records	8	6	2	0	1	1	5	2	3	1	10	3	14
High Use	14	19	10	2	6	5	3	2	5	8	10	15	33
72 Hrs	67	57	22	14	20	11	25	13	19	41	41	42	124
De facto	6	20	13	7	3	0	0	2	1	13	5	8	26

Figure 3.2 Breakdown of Coding Framework for Section 5(2)

Figure 3.2 above details the current coding for Section 5(2). The first row gives the total number of instances in reports where concerns in regard to this section are expressed and the following rows provide information on the breakdown of these instances in the current coding framework.

The Commission's Hospital Profile Statistics provide information on the use of Section 5(2) across the country and it is noted in the Commission's Seventh and Eighth Biennial Reports that the use of this Section has increased over the sampling period.

That this data is recorded via the Hospital Profile Statistics may account for both the relative lack of the recording of the High Use of this Section in reports and the concentration upon patients being detained for more than 72 hours (including where the Section has been allowed to lapse) and where patients are in effect de facto detained due references directing the implementation of Section 5(4) should they try to leave a ward.

This is however unlikely, particularly as the Commission undertook to more closely monitor the use of this Section after it first noted an increase in its use in the Sixth Biennial Report. It therefore may be concluded that either the current coding of this topic is incorrect or that the visiting Commissioners were not discussing the use of this Section on visits to Trusts to an extent justified by the increasing use of this Section.

There appears to have been a small drop of instances where patients have not been assessed within 72 hours (including where it has been allowed to lapse), and where it is noted that the Trust's records relating to the use, or its Audit of the use, of this Section are incomplete. This may be in part attributed to the Commission's practice of encouraging Trusts to audit the use of the Section where such instances of poor practice are noted.

Consent to Treatment (Forms 38 and 39)

Consent to Treatment issues are of significant interest to the Commission. Establishing that a patient has indeed agreed or can agree to medication which is accurately and clearly recorded is an area that the Commission must examine to ensure it fulfils its responsibilities under the Act.

Data were extracted from reports except in instances where there is not a record of the RMO recording the patient's capacity to consent or this record giving insufficient discussion of the patient's capacity to consent; along with instances where patients with a current Form 38 either appear to Commissioners incapable of giving consent or patients inform Commissioners that they are not complying with their medication.

The data suggested that the following issues may be of concern and needed more attention by the Commission:

1. recording of the discussion between the patient and RMO where consent is obtained;

2. the contacting of Second Opinion Appointed Doctors where a patient refuses or is incapable to consent after the initial three-month period;
3. the recording medication by the RMO on consent forms;
4. the attachment of the form to patients' medicine card for easy checking by staff;
5. the reviewing of forms on an annual basis or when a new RMO takes over the care of a detained patient.

The increased frequency of instances of concern relating to the recording of the discussion between the RMO and patient in which consent was obtained can be attributed to Forms 38 being included in the Commission's MRPA. The Eighth Biennial Report (p.169) highlights that nearly half of the Forms 38 examined as part of the Commission's MRPA (n=789) showed no record of the discussion between patients and the Registered Medical Officer (n= .386).

In both its Seventh and Eighth Biennial Reports the Commission documents its concerns in regards to the reviewing of consent after a year or where a new RMO takes over the responsibility of a patient's treatment plan. The examination of the Forms 38 included in the MRPA show that "a small but significant proportion (7 per cent) of Forms 38 had not been signed by the current RMO and 72 (9 per cent) were over a year old." This is slightly less than the number of instances in the sample – 18 per cent.

In 24 per cent the instances of concern relate to patients who are receiving medication either not authorised on their Form 38 or doses over that stated on the Form 38. Twenty-one per cent of instances relate to patients having no Form 38 or 39 when the three-month limit has been exceeded. In both these cases patients are receiving medication illegally. Twenty-one per cent of instances refer to the relevant forms of patients not being attached to medicine cards.

The Commission has concerns in regard to the recording and authorisation of Forms 38 – by BNF categories, dose-ranges and the Routes of Administration – and has advised the Secretary of State of the need to include such advice in the revision of the Code of Practice. This now states that medication should be documented "by name or, ensuring that the number of drugs authorised in each class is indicated, by the classes described in the British National Formulary" (16.14). It appears that these concerns are justified with 380 of the 539 instances (70 per cent) of concern in reports relating to the completion of the forms in this regard.

The breakdown of Forms 38 and 39 issues can be found in Figure 7 on page 36 of the report. It can be clearly seen here that the Commission is finding deficiencies in Forms 38 and 39 on 68 per cent of all visiting data available in the sample. This is a matter that needs further investigation, as it appears to show a lack of influence in regard to improving practice. When the second stage of analysis is completed, the Trusts in the sample which show persistent problems for Forms 38 and 39 will be known. It is intended that this data will be forwarded to the Commission for their information.

Section 17

The breakdown of Section 17 Leave by Mini Indicators can be found in Figure 8 on page 36 of the report.

Concern over poor practice in regard to the recording and authorising of leave can be found in the Commission's Sixth, Seventh and Eighth Biennial Reports on page 100, page 51 and page 92 respectively and the first National Visit on page 9. The sampled data confirm that the majority of concerns with this Section surround the completion and authorisation of forms (78 per cent; n=344).

This figure, along with the apparent lack of giving copies to a patient's nearest relative (n=64) or such relatives acting as escorts for patients without the proper authorisation of the hospital managers (n=19), Home Office approval for leave being unavailable on the day of the visit (n=22), and the poor design of leave forms (n=84) indicates that the Commission is frequently finding that Trusts are having difficulty in ensuring good practice in documenting leave.

As with Forms 38 and 39, it is expected that Trusts which have persistent poor practice in regard to Section 17 will be forwarded to the Commission for their information.

Topics Included in the Commission's "Matters Requiring Particular Attention" (MRPA)

Though Form 38 (Consent to Treatment) forms part of the Commission's MRPA, the review of these forms is an essential part of the examination of detained patients' statutory documentation undertaken on visits. Consequently, they are excluded from this section for the sake of convenience.

The Physical Examination and the Ethnic Monitoring of detained patients have been coded.

An important point to note is that issues included in the MRPA are recorded on a distinct form during visits and so it is possible that the topics may be discussed at the final meeting held at the conclusion of a visit but not be included in the Commission's report. This, in particular, may be the case in regard to the recording of ethnicity as the Commission additionally collects this information via its meetings with detained patients' record.

This said, it was expected that all MRPA topics including Form 38 would have an increased presence in reports during Period Two of the sample in comparison with Period One. The initial frequency analysis confirms this is indeed the case.

The Physical Examination of Patients

As the Commission's Eighth Biennial Report notes, research shows that detained patients, particularly long-term patients, have an increased likelihood of suffering from physical ailments.

Of the 789 visits examined, 99 instances of poor practice in regard to the coding issues above occurred. Eighty-three references were made concerning the lack of recording the undertaking and/or reviewing of a physical examination of some or most detained patients. Thirty-eight instances referred to the apparent lack of a specific Protocol, the Protocol being insufficient in regard to recording and/or the reviewing of physical examinations, or staff being unable to produce a Protocol when asked.

In the Eighth Biennial Report, the Commission discusses the results of its initial analysis of data collected concerning its MRPA. Here, the results of its collection of data of over 1,200 wards show a relatively high instance of Trusts' protocols not clearly specifying the need to review the examination of patients at least annually (56 per cent). Of the 80 per cent of the wards with detained patients resident for over a month, 23 per cent did not have a full record of the undertaking of an examination for the most recently detained patient. While, of the 48 per cent of the wards with detained patients resident for over a year, 47 per cent could not produce records relating to review examinations of long-stay detained patients' physical health.

The Commission notes that these figures, as with the coding undertaken for this project, relate to the recording of the undertaking and reviewing of physical examinations; not that they have not being undertaken. The physical examination of a patient once he or she is detained can be seen as an integral part of the care process started upon admission. Consequently a protocol to provide guidance to staff is unnecessary. However, like the Commission, the project teams held the view that recording the physical wellbeing or otherwise of detained patients is of considerable importance in providing the delivery of patient-centred care.

Ethnic Monitoring

The Commission discusses the provision of services for ethnic minority groups in its Biennial Reports. The concerns expressed by the Commission in its visit reports regarding the meeting of the Race and Culture needs of detained patients is a topic remaining to be analysed. However, the recording of ethnicity is part of the MRPA, and analysis in this respect has been completed as far as currently possible.

The recording of patients' ethnicity upon admission became a mandatory requirement in April 1995 (EL (94) 77). The Commission rightly is concerned with this issue, as inadequate recording will hamper its own ability to monitor the rights and interests of detained patients from ethnic minorities. Consequently this must be the case for Trusts also. In the Seventh Biennial Report it is noted that the implementation of ethnic monitoring has been slow and consequently data made available to Commissioners on visits had been "very patchy and ad hoc."

The Commission's central concern in regard to ethnic monitoring is that it is recorded at ward level so staff are aware of patients' needs; and that it is recorded using the ONS categories.

Of the 789 visits, 121 instances of poor practice were found to be present in Commission reports. As noted in Figure 10 on page 36, 17 instances were in Period One and 104 in Period Two. This means that 23 per cent of the visit reports in Period Two contain instances were the Commission expresses its concern regarding the recording of ethnicity.

The coding for ethnicity concerns the lack of ethnic recording and inconsistent use of ONS categories at ward level within Trusts. The Commission's MRPA data shows that 38 per cent of ward notes (n=1276) did not record ethnicity and the recording of ethnicity for 25 per cent of hospitals did not comply with ONS categories. Clearly this data along with that extracted from reports for this project illustrates that Trusts need to be vigilant in ensuring all information concerning their detained patients is adequately recorded so it can be utilised as an indirect tool by which to respond to the cultural diversity of service users. The new Code of Practice states that data should be obtained by sex and race concerning compulsory admissions and it is hoped the Commission will be able to report an improvement in practice in its next Biennial Report as a consequence of this new guidance.

Physical Examinations and Ethnic Monitoring

Upon initial analysis it appears that the CVT One and Two areas – Anglia & East Thames and Oxford & NW Thames respectively – have a considerably higher frequency of problems in the recording of ethnicity and physical examinations than other CVT areas. This information would be invaluable to the Commission if it were the case, particularly as it would enable resources to be better targeted to monitor the two topics within these CVT areas.

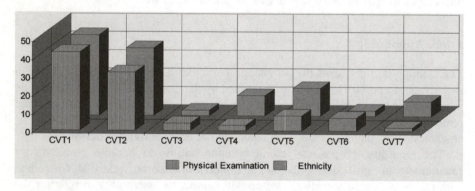

Figure 3.3 Physical Examination and Recording of Ethnicity

However other possibilities exist due to the topics being part of the MRPA. It may be that these figures reflect Commissioner practice to record these issues in reports as well as on the MRPA forms for these CVT areas as opposed to others. Or that the MRPA forms have been completed with a higher frequency in these areas when compared with the others, and so Commissioners are more aware of the need to record these issues in reports.

It would seem reasonable for the Commission to explore its MRPA data set to see if similar findings to this project occur or, if it indeed is the case that more MRPA forms were returned for CVT Two and Three than for other CVTs. If this latter option is the case then a tentative conclusion can be made that these topics are more frequently mentioned in reports in CVT Two and Three due to the higher use of the MRPA forms.

Section 132

Section 132 of the Act requires hospitals to inform patients of their rights. In its Eighth Biennial Report the Commission notes that the recording of the giving and of rights has improved, particularly in respect to the recording of patients' understanding of their rights – a concern noted in the Seventh Biennial Report. As the current data set has missing data in Period One, it is not possible to currently comment upon the data in this respect.

Currently, instances of concern in regard to the recording of the giving and reviewing of patients' rights occur in 22 per cent of the data set (n=171).

Topics Mainly Found on Full and Joint Visits

The availability of Section 12 Doctors and the Place of Safety under Section 136 are topics included mainly in Full and Joint Visits. Though visits to Social Service Departments only also include these topics it is not expected that the data consequently lost will make any findings inconclusive. For example, of the 220 visits in the sample, concerns in regard to these topics occur 46 per cent and 43 per cent respectively. This of course presumes that these topics where discussed in visits only in the sampled data – which is not necessarily the case. However these figures give an indication that the exclusion of Social Service Department visits has not affected the frequency of concerns – particularly as the availability of Section 12 Doctors is known to be a national concern.

Trust Response to Commission Reports

Trust Responses to Instances of Issues of Concern in Reports

In total there are 1,757 instances of concern for all the topics. Figure 3.4 shows the breakdown of the response by Trusts to these instances. It illustrates that the vast majority of responses are positive, i.e. the Trust in question agrees to undertake an Audit of its use of Section 5(4) or review its Section 17 Forms. Missing data – where responses by Trust are missing – totals 5 per cent. Trust replies that do not contain a response to the issue highlighted in the Commission report stand at 2 per cent, while instances of the Trust informing the Commission it has made a mistake (i.e. ethnic monitoring is indeed recorded on patient sheets) total 2 per cent. The number of instances that Trusts disagree with either the Commission's findings or recommendations is 2 per cent (i.e. a patient's Form 38 was indeed present on the ward during the visit). As quoted from the reports:

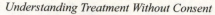
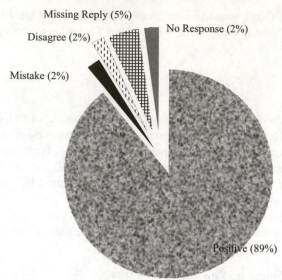

Missing Reply (5%)

No Response (2%)

Disagree (2%)

Mistake (2%)

Positive (89%)

Figure 3.4 Breakdown of the Response by Trusts to Instances of Concern

The Trust shares the Commissioners' concerns about the lack of records of physical examinations for all patients. 'Dr Jones' has written to all medical staff reminding them of this requirement, and will ensure that this policy is audited.

The Mental Health Unit does not have a formal policy on the physical examination of patients. The view of the senior medical staff is that all patients are subject to a physical examination on admission and during the patient's stay if signs and symptoms occur which require further investigation.

Although the Commissioners reported that ethnic origin is not recorded in the ward notes, this is in fact not the case as the information is recorded in the summary at the front of the notes.

Positive replies do not mean an issue has been remedied to the satisfaction of Commissioners. It is possible for a Trust to constantly give a positive response and still on all visits undertaken to it the same topic of concern is mentioned in reports (i.e. the persistent lack of Section 12 Doctors). However the number of positive responses would seem to suggest at this stage that a good working relationship exists between Trusts and the Commission, with the findings of the Commission being accepted and an appropriate course of action agreed by Trusts via its response.

The hope is that this chapter provides a little insight into the visiting activities of the Commission and the ways in which data are collected and find their way into the biennial reports.

Chapter 4

The Reform of the Mental Health Act

Jeffrey Cohen

The Drivers for Change

Just 10 years after the passing of the 1983 Mental Health Act, the Mental Health Act Commission, in its Fifth Biennial Report, was urging that "a full review of the 1983 Act is now needed." Again, in its Seventh Report, the Commission pointed to increasing difficulties in the application and interpretation of parts of the legislation, which did not correspond to how services were being delivered. Mental health services were changing from being primarily hospital based to more of a community focus and these changes were not reflected in the legislative framework. The Mental Health Act 1983, the origins of which lay in the 1959 Act, was essentially about hospital treatment and had become out of date.

The Government was also under mounting pressure to respond to demands for greater protection of the public following a small number of homicides committed by mentally-disordered individuals who had been discharged to the community. Although such incidents are rare, particularly stranger homicides,[1] media coverage has led to a distorted perception that people with a mental disorder are dangerous. Two cases involving the unprovoked killing of strangers typify the fears. In one case, Christopher Clunis, who was well known to mental health services and had been diagnosed with paranoid schizophrenia, killed Jonathan Zito on a railway platform in 1992. The subsequent inquiry exposed a catalogue of failure in the co-ordination of his care in the community and a shameful lack of follow-up to ensure he received medical treatment. In 1995, the Government introduced some measures in an attempt to tighten up compliance with treatment in the community, including a Supervision Register to keep track of high risk patients and Supervised Discharge to ensure that such patients received after-care services following discharge from detention under the Mental Health Act. However, these measures stopped short of actual compulsory treatment in the community on account of a misguided view at that time, that this would contravene the European Convention of Human Rights. The second case was that of Michael Stone, who was convicted of the homicide of a mother and daughter and seriously injuring a second daughter, in broad daylight, in a peaceful country lane in South East England in 1996. He had previously been detained on the grounds of psychopathic disorder, but it was mistakenly reported at the time that he had been

---

1 According to the National Confidential Inquiry into Suicide and Homicide 2001 Report "Safety First", 9 per cent of homicides in England and Wales had been in contact with mental health services in the year before the offence. Furthermore, mentally-ill perpetrators were less likely to kill a stranger than those without mental illness.

refused re-admission to hospital because he was considered untreatable.[2] This case prompted the Government to consider introducing legislation which would limit the discretion of psychiatrists on the use of detention for individuals described as being 'dangerous and with a severe personality disorder', whether or not they could benefit from treatment and whether or not they had been convicted of a crime. It was estimated that there were between 2,000 and 2,500 such people of whom about 700 were living in the community, the rest being in prison or secure hospitals.[3]

We have seen in the earlier chapters of this book that throughout the history of mental health services there has been a tension between ensuring that people with mental disorder receive care and treatment, if necessary without their consent, for their own health or safety or the protection of others and the right of the individual not to be unjustly deprived of his or her liberty, nor to be subject to the abuse or misuse of professional power. Accordingly, another driver for change has been to ensure that adequate safeguards are in place to protect the human rights of those who are or may become subject to compulsory powers for reasons of mental disorder.

There has been a series of challenges where the compatibility of the Mental Health Act with the European Convention of Human Rights (ECHR) has been called into question. These have increased in frequency since the ECHR was incorporated into British law in October 2000 following the Human Rights Act 1998. In some cases it has been possible for the courts to interpret the Mental Health Act in a way which makes it compatible with the ECHR. So as not to compromise the right to privacy and a family life under Article 8 of the ECHR, the courts have stretched the meaning of the statutory language so that Approved Social Workers (ASWs) can be more flexible in whom they consult as Nearest Relative prior to applying for admission under Section 3 of the Mental Health Act. ASWs can consult with the same sex partner of a patient as though they were living together as husband and wife[4] and the statutory requirement to consult with the Nearest Relative unless it is 'not reasonably practicable' no longer obliges the ASW to consult with a Nearest Relative where there would be adverse consequences for the patient.[5] In other cases, it has been possible for the Government to ensure compliance with the ECHR by improving procedures. It has speeded up access to tribunals following a successful challenge against inordinate delays between an application and a hearing, which contravened ECHR Article 5(4) right for a speedy determination of the lawfulness

---

2   The subsequent inquiry (Report of the Independent Inquiry into the Care and Treatment of Michael Stone), which was not published, by the South East Coast Strategic Health Authority until September 2006, found that there was no evidence that the local forensic unit was unwilling to consider admitting Michael Stone. Unfortunately, the Unit were denied the chance to make a fully informed decision about admission shortly before the murder by an inadequate communication from a general practitioner.

3   Home Office and Department of Health (1999) Managing Dangerous People with Severe Personality Disorder, *Proposals for Policy Development*, London: HO/DoH.

4   R (on the application of SSG) vs Liverpool City Council, the Secretary of State for Health and LS (Interested Party), October 22, 2002.

5   R (on the application of E) vs Bristol City Council (Administrative Court, 2005).

of detention.[6] Following another successful challenge[7] in which the court made a declaration of incompatibility with the Article 5 right to liberty, the Government issued a Remedial Order to change the wording of the Mental Health Act 1983. This switched the burden of proof so that the hospital authority must satisfy the tribunal that a patient should continue to be detained rather than the patient having to prove that the criteria justifying his or her detention no longer exist.

However, a number of human rights issues remained unresolved. Lord Steyn identified what came to be known as the Bournewood gap when describing an "indefensible gap in our mental health law."[8] He was referring to the position of compliant incapacitated patients who can be admitted to hospital without the formality of the Mental Health Act and without any of the consequent safeguards to protect the patient from professional misjudgement and the arbitrary deprivation of liberty. Where a patient does not have mental capacity to take decisions about medical treatment and where in the doctor's opinion such treatment is in the patient's best interests, a doctor is entitled to treat without the patient's consent, provided in the case of mental disorder the patient does not object. If a patient is incapable and does not object, he or she can be treated under the Common Law principle of necessity. In the Bournewood case, the patient, HL, was informally admitted to a psychiatric hospital and removed from the care of his carers in the face of strong opposition from them. HL was a 48 year old autistic man, who was unable to speak. He did not attempt to leave hospital but, had he done so, the psychiatrist in charge of his treatment would have prevented him. The House of Lords decided that this position was in accordance with the Mental Health Act, although in the words of Lord Steyn "effective and unqualified control" was placed "in the hands of the hospital psychiatrist and other healthcare professionals." Eventually, the case reached the European Court of Human Rights in Strasbourg, which found that HL's stay in hospital did amount to detention, that it was not in accordance with a procedure prescribed by law, as required by Article 5(1) pf the ECHR and that he was denied the right under Article 5(4) to have his detention reviewed by a court.[9] There could be as many as 48,000 incapacitated patients who are de facto detained in hospital in any one year[10] and many more residents in a similar position in nursing and residential care homes. It became incumbent on the Government to find a legislative framework which will bridge the human rights gap in mental health law exposed by the Bournewood case.

The main effect of the European ruling in the Bournewood case is that, if the circumstances of an incapable patient's admission to hospital amounts to a deprivation of liberty, it would contravene the ECHR to continue treatment on an informal basis and an application should be considered for admission under Section 2 or 3 of the

---

6   R (on the application of KB and others) vs Mental Health Review Tribunal and the Secretary of State for Health [2002] EWHC 639.

7   H vs MHRT (South East and London Region) [2000].

8   R vs Bournewood Community and Mental Health NHS Trust, ex parte L [1999] AC 458.

9   HL vs The United Kingdom (Application no. 45508/99), Judgment 5th October 2004.

10 Mental Health Act Commission (1998), written submission to the House of Lords, following the Court of Appeal decision in December 1997 that HL had been unlawfully detained.

Mental Health Act. However, incapable patients are at a further disadvantage if they also lack the capacity to exercise the right to make an application to the tribunal. For patients detained under Section 2, there is no automatic referral to a tribunal and for those under Section 3 an automatic referral only takes place if detention is continued beyond the first six months. Thus the incompetent patient does not have the same protection within the provisions of the Mental Health Act as the competent patient. The Court of Appeal did declare, in the case of an incapacitated patient subject to Section 2 that the lack of an automatic referral to a tribunal was incompatible with the European Convention of Human Rights. However, the declaration was overturned by the House of Lords in that the right to information under Section 132 of the Act is designed to facilitate access to a tribunal. In addition, the Secretary of State can be asked to exercise his or her power to refer a case to the tribunal at any time.[11]

There is an argument that these pressures for change could be dealt with satisfactorily within the existing legislative framework and that the objectives of the Government could be achieved without the need for a completely new Mental Health Act. As we have seen above, either the Government has been able to amend the current legislation, for example with the introduction of a Remedial Order, or the courts have been able to interpret the Mental Health Act in such a way, as with the Nearest Relative cases, so as to accommodate human rights' concerns. The courts have also interpreted other provisions of the Mental Health Act to bring its implementation in line with current practice. With regard to community treatment, Section 17 of the 1983 Act, which enables the Responsible Medical Officer to authorise leave from hospital, can now be used as a mechanism to require the patient to continue to accept medical treatment whilst in the community for extended periods. It had been understood since the Hallstrom Judgment in 1985 that a patient could only be detained under the Act if there was a genuine need for detention in hospital.[12] It was unlawful to renew a patient's liability to detention under Section 3 if he or she was on leave and not actually receiving 'treatment in hospital', thereby keeping the patient on what had been termed 'the long leash'. However, in the case of DR,[13] the Judge, Wilson J., considerably widened the definition of 'treatment in hospital', famously declaring "there is no magic in a bed." Liability for detention can continue, provided there is a significant component in the care and treatment plan, which necessitates the patient to attend hospital (for example, for a multi-disciplinary review of progress). In the later CS case,[14] a four-weekly ward round and weekly sessions with the ward psychologist as part of a programme of transition from hospital to community based care was held to justify continued liability to detention. The judge described the in-hospital treatment as "gossamer thin," but sufficient.

In similar fashion, the courts have interpreted the 'treatability criteria' so widely that it could possibly obviate the need for the Government to bring in legislation to ensure that those with personality disorder come within its provisions. Under the 1983 Act, a patient cannot be detained under the categories of mental impairment or psychopathic disorder unless the treatability criteria are satisfied; i.e. the mental

---

11 MH vs Secretary of State for Health and others [2005], UKHL 60.

12 R vs Hallstrom ex p W (No 2); R V Gardner ex p L [1986].

13 R (on the application of D.R.) vs Mersey Care NHS Trust [2002].

14 R (CS) vs MHRT [2004].

disorder can either be alleviated or prevented from deterioration. There is no need for there to be positive clinical measures to satisfy these criteria. The House of Lords has held that a patient may be detained even if it is only his symptoms – and not the mental disorder – that can be managed. It is sufficient, for example, for a patient categorised with psychopathic disorder to be merely contained in a safe environment as a means of managing his anger.[15]

The Review of the Mental Health Act

When the Government announced its 'root and branch review' of the mental health legislation in September 1998, they would not have foreseen the difficulties in bringing about new legislation. The reform of the Mental Health Act was one of the main planks in its vision for the modernisation of mental health services, as Frank Dobson, as Secretary of State for Health wrote,

> We are going to bring the law on mental health up-to-date. In particular to ensure that patients who might otherwise be a danger to themselves and others are no longer allowed to refuse to comply with the treatment they need. We will also be changing the law to permit the detention of a small group of people who have not committed a crime but whose untreatable psychiatric disorder makes them dangerous. The law will be changed to deliver this protection for the public while at the same time respecting the civil rights of patients.[16]

Legislative reform timeline	
October 1998	Expert committee established
July 1999	Consultation paper "Managing Dangerous People with Severe Personality Disorder" published
November 1999	Expert Committee Report "Review of the Mental Health Act 1983" published
	Green Paper "Reform of the Mental Health Act 1983" published
December 2000	White Paper, "Reforming the Mental Health Act" published
June 2002	Draft Mental Health Bill published for consultation
September 2004	New draft of Mental Health Bill published
March 2005	Report of Joint Committee on draft Mental Health Bill published
May 2005	Mental Health Bill listed in Queen's Speech
July 2005	Government response to the report of the Joint Committee on the draft Mental Health Bill
March 2006	Government abandon the Bill to reform the Mental Health Act and announce proposals to amend the 1983 Mental Health Act
November 2006	Health Bill to amend the 1983 Mental Health Act introduced in the House of Lords
July 2007	Mental Health Act 2007 received royal assent

---

15 Reid vs Secretary of State for Scotland [1999].

16 Department of Health (1998), "Foreword by the Secretary of State" in *Modernising Mental Health Services. Safe, Sound and Supportive.*

The Expert Committee, chaired by Genevra Richardson, was commissioned to advise on how mental health legislation should be shaped to reflect contemporary patterns of care within a framework which balances the need to protect the rights of individual patients and the need to ensure public safety. They were expected to report speedily. Paul Boateng, then Minister of State for Health, told them that "we do not have time to spend in years of contemplation." He did not achieve his objective.

The Expert Committee published its review in July 1999.[17] Their recommendations were founded on two basic principles: 'non-discrimination' and 'patient autonomy'. By non-discrimination, the Committee meant that "wherever possible, the principles governing mental health care should be the same as those governing physical health care." This, the Committee stated, inevitably leads to an emphasis on 'patient autonomy' – the freedom for those with capacity to make their own treatment choice. A capable patient has an absolute right to refuse treatment for a physical disorder for any reason, whatever the consequences, even when the decision may lead to his or her own death. Applying the same principles to treatment for mental disorder, the Mental Health Act would authorise treatment in the absence of consent only to those who lack capacity. However, the Committee recognised that there was a difficulty in applying these principles to those with capacity who present a danger either to themselves or, even more so, to others. Where there was a serious risk to others, as in the case of some people with psychopathic disorder, the Committee favoured a pragmatic approach which would allow compulsory intervention despite the inconsistency with the principle of autonomy. They were uncertain about whether such an exception should be extended to protect patients with capacity from committing suicide or inflicting serious harm on themselves, which was, in the view of the committee, a matter of moral choice for politicians to consider. The key concern of the Committee was to ensure that any infringement of patient autonomy was properly considered and justified.

The Government, in its Green Paper, published in November 1999,[18] rejected the Richardson Committee's capacity model for the use of compulsion and put forward a risk model.

> It is the degree of risk that patients with mental disorder pose, to themselves or others, that is crucial … Questions of capacity – while still relevant to the plan of care and treatment – may be largely irrelevant to the question of whether or not a compulsory order should be made.

The Government had already separately published proposals for managing dangerous people with severe personality disorder, which controversially advocated changes in legislation for the detention of such individuals on the basis of the risk they present, even if they were not treatable and, if necessary, for an indefinite period.[19]

---

17 Department of Health (1999), Review of the Expert Committee: Review of the Mental Health Act 1983, Cm 4480, London: DoH.

18 Department of Health (1999), *Reform of the Mental Health Act 1983*, Proposals for Consultation, Cm 4480, London: DoH.

19 Home Office and Department of Health (1999), op cit.

On 20 December 2000 the White Paper was published.[20] This proposed a single route to compulsion which comprised of three stages – a preliminary assessment by three mental health professionals; formal assessment and initial treatment under compulsory powers for up to 28 days; and longer term compulsion, for which authorisation by a tribunal was required.

There would be a new broad definition of mental disorder covering "any disability or disorder of mind or brain, whether permanent or temporary, which results in an impairment or disturbance of mental functioning." The wide discretion afforded to doctors in this broadly drawn definition of mental disorder would be limited by the requirement that the mental disorder must be sufficiently serious to warrant specialist mental health intervention and without which the patient would be likely to be at risk of serious harm, including deterioration in health, or to pose a significant risk of serious harm to other people. Care and treatment beyond 28 days would be specified in a care plan, which would have to be authorised by the Tribunal. Where compulsion was in the patient's own best interests, the care plan would have to be of "direct therapeutic benefit." Where compulsion was because of risk to others, the plan must be "necessary directly to treat the underlying mental disorder and/or to manage the behaviours arising from it." The objective of this last proposal was to replace the notion of treatability so as to bring dangerous people with personality disorder within the provisions of the Mental Health Act without the need for separate legal provisions. Thus, a psychiatrist would be less able to refuse to treat patients with personality disorder by declaring them untreatable.

The tribunal would specify whether the patient was to be detained in a particular location (i.e. a hospital); or, if not detained (i.e. subject to compulsory treatment in the community) the consequences of non-compliance.

The White Paper announced a series of new safeguards for mentally disordered patients who lacked capacity but were compliant and so could not be made subject to the compulsory provisions of the Mental Health Act. Incapacitated patients, who were 'de facto' detained would have a right of appeal to a tribunal. A clinical supervisor would be required to prepare a care plan and for this to be examined by a Second Opinion Doctor. They would also fall within the remit of the Commission for Mental Health. The Commission for Mental Health itself would lose the responsibility for regular visiting, but it was to be given new responsibilities for collecting and analysing information, overseeing standards of specialist advocacy (to which patients subject to compulsion would have a new right of access) and the training of professionals with key roles under the new legislation.

The White Paper represented a shift back towards a more legalistic approach by enhancing the role of the tribunal in the authorisation of compulsion beyond 28 days. Throughout the last two centuries in the history of mental health legislation, the medical and legal approaches have competed for dominance. The apotheosis of the legal approach was the Lunacy Act 1890, which imposed rigid procedures and criteria for compulsory admission. Orders for commitment had to be made by magistrates and only people with the most severe mental illness were likely to be admitted. The 1959 Mental Health Act marked a significant shift towards the medical approach.

---

20 Department of Health and Home Office (2000), *Reforming the Mental Health Act Part 1: The New Legal Framework and Part II: High-risk Patients*, Cm 5016, London: DoH/HO.

It established that admission to psychiatric hospital should usually take place on an informal basis, but where compulsion was still necessary the decision to use powers of detention became a medical rather than a judicial one. The framework of the 1959 Act was largely followed by the 1983 Act, with some additional legal safeguards to limit professional discretion and enhance the rights of detained patients.

There was substantial opposition to the White Paper proposals. A Mental Health Alliance was formed in 1999 (consisting of mental health professional groups, user groups, lawyers, voluntary associations, research bodies and carers' associations) uniquely working together for the sole purpose of improving mental health legislation. The very existence of this group is testament to the changes that have occurred in the strength of the mental health lobby. It is unimaginable, for example that, in 1959 or even in 1983, such diverse interest groups could have campaigned together under the same banner.

Despite the greater emphasis on a legal model, the main thrust of the criticisms of the legislative proposals was that the legal criteria for the use of compulsion had not been made restrictive enough. There were three main areas of concern. One was that the broadening of the definition of mental disorder would bring a wider range of people within the ambit of mental health legislation, including people with learning disability, those who misuse substances and those who are considered to be sexually deviant. The second was the breaking of the link with treatability, which would make it possible to detain people with personality disorder for indefinite periods mainly for the purpose of social control rather than any benefit to the individual patient. The third was the introduction of compulsory treatment in the community, which would give rise to concerns that there could be resistance to seeking psychiatric help from users who fear that they may be made subject to compulsion if they disagree with the treatment recommended by the psychiatrist.

Following the substantial criticisms from many of the major stakeholders, the pace of change slowed down. A draft Mental Health Bill was not released until June 2002,[21] 18 months after the White Paper. The draft Bill did not address the concerns which had been raised and, in some respects, took a step in the opposite direction. The broad definition of mental disorder was still not circumscribed narrowly enough by other criteria to limit the use of compulsion and the link between the mental disorder and its treatability was loosened even further. The requirement that there should be treatment for the underlying disorder and/or the management of behaviours arising from it was replaced by the vague condition that "appropriate medical treatment for the mental disorder is available in the patient's case." Furthermore patients who posed a substantial risk of serious harm to others (i.e. dangerous people with severe personality disorder), would be exempted from the requirement that compulsion be used only if treatment cannot be provided in any other way. In other words, the principle of the 'least restrictive alternative' would not apply to this group of patients, who could be subject to indefinite detention even if there was no direct benefit to them.

The draft Bill also abandoned the White Paper proposal to replace the Mental Health Act Commission with another independent body. Instead, its functions would

---

21 Department of Health (2002), *Draft Mental Health Bill*, Cm 5538 – I. The Bill was accompanied by two associated documents: The Draft Mental Health Bill Explanatory Notes, Cm 5538-II and Mental Health Bill Consultation Document, CM 5538-III.

be somewhat diluted and be carried out by the Commission for Health Audit and Improvement (later known as the Healthcare Commission) with only a limited power to visit local services. The loss of a body dedicated to keep the mental health legislation under review could significantly weaken the safeguards against the abuse of the power of compulsion. This is a particular concern given that compulsion might potentially be extended to a wider range of people and would be available in the community as well as the hospital.

The opposition of the Mental Health Alliance was as strong as ever. The Government intended to announce the introduction of the Bill in the Queen's Speech in November 2002, but decided to withdraw it from its legislative programme to give more time to reflect on the criticisms. Neither did it appear a year later in 2003. Instead, the Government eventually introduced a second draft Mental Health Bill in September 2004 and submitted it to parliamentary scrutiny.

The Second Draft Bill

The Joint Parliamentary Committee on the draft Mental Health Bill published its report on 23 March 2005. Its purpose was to scrutinise the second draft Bill and, on the basis of consultation, recommend improvements before a Bill proper was introduced into Parliament. It consulted widely with all the key stakeholders, including professionals, service users and carers and published the oral evidence together with some of the written evidence in a second volume, alongside its main report.[22] One consideration was whether the Government should proceed with the Bill at all, given the level of opposition to some of its key clauses and given, as discussed above, that existing legislation can be interpreted and adapted to meet, at least to some degree, the objectives of the Government. On balance, the joint committee accepted that "it is desirable for thorough legislative reform to be implemented ... to set important aspects of mental health policy on a new course for the next 20 years or so."

Genevra Richardson, herself, accepted that the basic structural reforms were there in the new Bill; as she said, in her evidence to the joint committee:

> In strictly formal terms, the Government seems to have accepted much of that institutional structure [i.e. that which was recommended by the Richardson Committee]. In the new Bill, you have got a single gateway to compulsory power, you have got a broad diagnostic definition and you have got early intervention of an independent decision maker in the shape of the Tribunal, and an agreed care plan.[23]

However, Professor Richardson and others were not happy with the Bill. The source of unhappiness was not just in the detail, but in some fundamental matters. These were in summary:

- the nature of the guiding principles underlying the legislation and whether or not they should appear on the face of the Bill;

---

22 Joint Committee on the Draft Mental Health Bill (2005), Volumes I and II, HL Paper 79-I and II; HC 95 – I and II.
23 Professor Genevra Richardson, Joint Committee Vol. II, evidence 2.

- the absence of exclusions linked to the broad definition of mental disorder to avoid certain groups being inappropriately caught in the mental health net;
- the width of the conditions which would set the threshold for the use of compulsion;
- the way in which the power of compulsory treatment in the community would be exercised; when, for whom and for how long;
- the interface between the legislation being introduced to provide a framework for people without capacity (the Capacity Act) and the Mental Health Bill;
- miscellaneous matters to do with resources, implementation and monitoring, including the abandonment of the successor body to the Mental Health Act Commission as a separate entity.

The Government retained the broad definition of mental disorder in the second draft Bill, although modifying it slightly to "an impairment of or disturbance in the functioning of the mind or brain resulting from any disability or disorder of the mind or brain."[24] The intention behind changing the wording of the definition around was to place the emphasis on the consequences rather than the cause of any mental disorder. Thus, it is not the diagnostic label itself that should be the determining factor in bringing people within the remit of the Bill, but the psychological dysfunction which results from it. The broad definition overcame the problem of the 1983 Act in which certain groups, which did not fall into any of the specified categories (namely mental illness, mental impairment, severe mental impairment or psychopathic disorder), such as those suffering from brain injury, were excluded from the treatment provisions of the Act. The disadvantage, of course, was that it was over-inclusive and drew within its scope people who behave in a deviant or anti-social way. As Dr Zigmund, on behalf of the Royal College of Psychiatrists, explained,

> We also need to be very careful that the mental health services do not become solely part of either the criminal justice system or an anti-social order system; that it has to be part of the health service. People who make lifestyle choices either to behave in a criminal manner, or to drink to excess, or to gamble, or to become addicted to cigarettes should not normally be forced to stop these by a health service.[25]

The Royal College's concerns derived from the Government's initial intention not to specify any exclusions from the coverage of the Bill. The 1959 and 1983 Acts made explicit exclusions so that no person could be made subject to the Act "by reason only of promiscuity or other immoral conduct, sexual deviancy or dependence on alcohol or drugs." The Government maintained that the exclusions were misunderstood or misapplied by mental health professionals. The presence of a drug or alcohol problem, even when presenting alongside a mental disorder, was sometimes used as grounds not to treat people, who were then denied the help they need.

Most witnesses providing evidence to the Parliamentary Committee were strongly in favour of keeping some exclusions. It was feared, without such exclusions, that the association of mental disorder with groups of anti-social offenders such as those

---

24 The definition in the first draft Bill was "any disability of disorder of mind or brain that results in an impairment or disturbance of mental functioning."

25 Royal College of Psychiatrists, Joint Committee Vol. II, evidence 79.

who sexually abuse children, would only serve to strengthen the link, in the public's mind, between mental health problems and criminal behaviour such as child abuse, further stigmatising all those with mental health problems.[26] On the other hand, there was an argument for removing the exclusions, as it would make services more accessible to mentally disordered offenders.[27] The Parliamentary Committee's view was that a broad definition of mental disorder needed to have clear exclusions so that the legislation could not be used as a means of social control. They recommended specific exclusions on the grounds of substance misuse, cultural or political beliefs or behaviours and sexual orientation, but not curiously on the grounds of sexual deviance. They believed that "it remains unclear whether some forms of non-violent and predatory behaviours may, in fact, be symptomatic of sexual disorder." The Government, in their response to the Joint Committee Report, relented with regard to those whose only mental disorder is dependency on alcohol or drugs. They conceded that an exclusion of some kind was desirable, provided that the presence of a drug or alcohol problem would not create any barrier to the proper use of compulsion for those with a 'dual diagnosis', including when a mental disorder arises out of, or is connected, with substance misuse.[28]

Clause 1 of the 2004 draft Bill specified that a Code of Practice must be published which would set out the general principles which should guide decisions made under the provisions of the Bill. These principles must be designed to ensure that:

- patients are involved in decisions affecting them;
- decisions are made fairly and openly;
- the least intrusive method of treatment is adopted and the restrictions imposed on patients are kept to the minimum necessary to protect their health or safety or to protect others.

The Government was initially opposed to setting out all the principles on the face of the Bill mainly because they wanted to retain some flexibility in the emphasis placed on certain principles, which would be easier to do within a Code of Practice. In particular, they had in mind the balance between the principles of maximising patient autonomy and the protection of the public, which may need to shift as practice developed over time. However, most witnesses giving evidence to the Joint Parliamentary Committee were strongly in favour of the principles being given statutory force. The Joint Parliamentary Committee itself believed it "essential that fundamental principles be set out on the face of the Bill" to make clear to practitioners working with the legislation on a daily basis what considerations should guide their actions.[29]

The Joint Committee commended the principles which appear on the face of the Mental Health (Care and Treatment) (Scotland) Act 2003. The Scottish Act does not include the contentious principles of patient autonomy and non-discrimination,

---

26 Mind, Joint Committee Vol. II, evidence 193.

27 Nacro, Joint Committee Vol. II, evidence 353.

28 Department of Health (2005), Government Response to the report of the joint committee on the draft Mental Health Bill, pp.11 and 12.

29 Joint Committee Vol. 1, p.24.

proposed by the Richardson Committee, underlying a pure capacity based model, but introduced a diluted version with the notion of 'significantly impaired decision-making'. Thus, in Scotland a patient cannot be made subject to compulsion unless his or her ability to make decisions about treatment is significantly impaired as a result of mental disorder. As a counter balance, the Joint Committee also recommended that the principles should be worded so as to reflect the need to protect the patient and others from harm.

The Government responded to the Joint Committee by repeating their view that it was possible that people may still retain the ability to make unimpaired decisions about their treatment even though they were at great risk to themselves or others. However, they were prepared to accept that principles should appear on the face of the Bill, provided that they could be drafted in a way which allowed for due protection to an individual's rights and autonomy, whilst also facilitating practitioners and others to take decisions that were necessary to minimise harm. The Government proposed that the principles should be broad and then considered in more detail in the Code of Practice and was also not in favour of a long list which would risk over-codification.

Clause 9 was the cornerstone of the Bill. It set out the conditions, all of which must be met before someone could be brought under formal powers. They were referred to as the relevant conditions and were as follows:

- The patient is suffering from a mental disorder.
- The mental disorder is of such a nature or degree as to warrant the provision of medical treatment.
- It is necessary that medical treatment be provided for the protection of the patient from suicide or serious self-harm or serious self-neglect of his/her health or safety, or for the protection of others.
- Medical treatment cannot be lawfully provided to the patient without him/ her being subject to the provisions of this Part of the Act. This condition does not apply to patients aged 16 or over who are at substantial risk of causing serious harm to others.
- Medical treatment is available which is appropriate to the patient's case, taking into account the nature or degree of the patient's mental disorder and all other circumstances of his/her case.

Clause 9 was the gateway into the use of compulsion. The five conditions determined who could be made subject to compulsion and in what circumstances. There were two underlying concerns about the nature of these conditions. One was that they were set too broadly and would result in an increase in the number of people made subject to compulsion. The other was that they were weighted too heavily towards the protection of the public rather than the treatment needs of the individual.

The number of people admitted under the Mental Health Act increased exponentially during the 1990s from just under 30,000 admissions in 1990 to a peak of 46,000 at the turn of the century, since when the numbers have levelled off.[30] The

---

30 Health and Social Care Information Centre (2005), Inpatients Formally Detained in Hospital under the Mental Health Act and Other Legislation, www.ic.nhs.uk.

reasons for the increase are varied. It could be a result of defensive practice in the context of a risk averse culture with mental health professionals erring on the side of safety by detaining people in hospital. It could be due to the revolving door patient; the pressure on the reducing number of beds leading to too early a discharge, relapse and re-admission. Rethink referred to the lack of preventative services, delays in accessing help for first time psychoses and that, for over 50 per cent, the first experience of treatment was detention. Use of the Act, they maintained, became the main rather than the last resort.[31] This certainly appeared to be the case for patients from African Caribbean and Black African Groups, whose over-representation in the numbers of people made subject to the Act amounted to five or six times what would be expected given their relative size in the population.[32]

There were two periods when there was a marked jump in the uses of the Act. One links to the publication of the second edition of the Code of Practice in 1993, which clarified that the grounds for compulsory admission could be satisfied for reasons of either health *or* safety alone, and not both health *and* safety, as had previously been the mistaken understanding. The second links to the Bournewood case and the intervening period in 1998 between the Court of Appeal and the House of Lords' decisions. The Court of Appeal court had ruled that incapacitated patients should be formally admitted, whether or not compliant, if the intention was not to allow them to leave the premises. The House of Lords reversed this decision, when they ruled that compliant incapacitated patients could be lawfully treated under the common law doctrine of necessity, without recourse to the Mental Health Act. These examples show the significance of the precise wording and interpretation of the conditions for compulsion for determining the number of patients who could potentially be made subject to the Act.

There were fears that the 'relevant conditions' set out in the draft Bill, the broad definition of mental disorder, the absence of exclusions, and the width of the other conditions would increase the use of compulsion still further. Under the 1983 Act, although the conditions might be even broader, the mental disorder had to be serious enough to justify admission to hospital. Under the draft Bill, the mental disorder only needed to be serious enough to justify treatment under a clinical supervisor. The need for a hospital bed was no longer a limiting factor.

The 1983 Act allowed mental health practitioners wide discretion in their use of their powers under the Act. The draft Bill limited discretion – if all the conditions were met, there was no choice but to use compulsion. Under the 1983 Act, Approved Social Workers only admitted about two-thirds of those who were referred for assessment. They were able to take into account 'all the circumstances' of the case. Consequently they could take into account factors not explicitly covered in the Act such as the capacity of the patient and whether existing care arrangements could meet the patient's needs; i.e. whether carers were able and willing to carry on. Thus, they could decide that the risk could be managed without compulsory admission to hospital, even though the criteria might have been satisfied.

In the absence of professional discretion, the other way to limit the use of compulsion was to narrow the conditions. The Government did this in the second draft

---

31 Rethink, Joint Committee Vol. II.
32 Mental Health Act Commission (1999), Eighth Biennial Report, p.237.

Bill by raising the threshold for admission for patients whose own health or safety was at risk. The conditions were significantly ratcheted up from the first draft Bill, which specified that compulsory powers had to be necessary simply on the grounds of the health or safety of the patient or the protection of others. The second draft Bill specified that medical treatment must be necessary for the protection of the patient from suicide or serious self harm or serious neglect of his health or safety or for the protection of others. Thus, risk to health was no longer sufficient on its own to justify the use of compulsion. However, there was no such limiting qualification relating to the condition of protection for others. The Government did not follow its own proposal in the White Paper, which specified that the risk to others had to be significant and the harm serious. The lack of any boundaries, some critics feared, could lead to compulsion being considered to cover protection from a minor nuisance.

The Government kept the special provision which appeared in the first draft Bill for those who presented a substantial risk of causing serious harm to others, allowing compulsion to be used even if the patient was willing to accept treatment. The intention was to enable mental health legislation to be used as a means of preventative detention for that group of people with a 'serious personality disorder' who might present dangers to the public, if they were free to leave hospital whenever they decided. However, the Government conceded, in their response to the Joint Committee, that there might be exceptional cases where high risk patients, who were compliant, might be treated without the use of compulsion.

The fifth condition concerning the availability of appropriate treatment was also targeted at ensuring those who presented a high risk were not excluded from being brought under compulsory powers. An attempt was made in the second draft Bill to soften the condition so that it was clear that there must be a holistic approach, which took account of all the patient's circumstances, ensuring that the care plan met the needs of the individual patient. However, it still fell short of incorporating the concept of therapeutic benefit and so did not satisfy the principle of reciprocity, that nobody should be compelled to accept treatment which was not of benefit to them.

A considerable number of stakeholders were alarmed by the disproportionate attention given to the small number of people who were deemed dangerous. The Mental Health Alliance believed that "while protection of others is a legitimate goal, the overemphasis is misplaced and will backfire and far from protecting public safety, it will undermine it." It perpetuated the perception in the public mind that people with a mental disorder were dangerous whereas there was only a modest increase in risk to others from people with a mental illness. It also led to unrealistic expectations about the prediction and elimination of risk. The outcome might be that, when incidents did occur, the confidence of and in experienced practitioners could be undermined. It reinforced the demand for a more coercive approach based more on a fear of failure than a genuine assessment of service user needs.

The Government have bridled at the criticism that they had given too much prominence to considerations of risk and protection of the public. They claimed that the majority of stakeholders represented health and social care professionals and service users. Few were from those with responsibility for protecting the public or the general public themselves. Although exaggerated by the media, the fact remained, the Government stated, "that there are significant numbers of homicides by mentally disordered people each year – some of which are preventable."[33] The Government's line was supported by those who argued that the 'treatability' clause in the 1983 Act has been used as a way of effectively refusing to offer services of any sort even on a consensual basis. Michael Howlett from the Zito Trust pointed out that, in 1984, 14 per cent of people with so-called psychopathic disorder were being treated in the NHS, but 10 years later the figure was under 3 per cent. Consequently, the Zito Trust concluded that the "treatability criterion as a loophole should be excluded from the current legislation so that people can be brought into the NHS and other services, having had an assessment of their needs."[34]

Another controversial issue concerned the use of compulsory treatment in the community. The draft Bill proposed the introduction of non-residential orders (NROs), whereby a non-resident patient could be required to attend at a specified place at specified times; reside at a specified place; make himself available for assessment during specified periods; and not engage in specified conduct. The Bill would not permit the forcible treatment of a patient outside of a hospital. If a patient failed to comply with treatment, then a clinical supervisor could decide that he or she should be admitted to hospital as a resident patient. The Government intended NROs to be targeted on revolving door patients, who had already been subject to frequent periods of treatment under compulsion. The case for community treatment was powerfully made by Jayne Zito, whose husband was killed by Christopher Clunis,

> … individuals like Christopher Clunis should not be hospitalised for a lifetime because of that profile [non-compliant with medication, transient and dangerous], they should have a right to live in our communities with appropriate support and with appropriate legislation to ensure that they take their treatment so that they can live safely within our communities.

The Mental Health Alliance was opposed to the introduction of NROs as drafted in the Bill. They identified a number of fears held by service users:

- NROs would increase the chances of being compulsorily detained if the service user disagreed with the treatment recommended by the psychiatrist.
- The element of control over home life would be an infringement of privacy.
- It would be difficult to come off an NRO, even if mental health improved, if the medical view was that treatment was preventing relapse.
- NROs were likely to be drug focused, as that is the only treatment which can be effectively enforced, even if the benefits are dubious. The number of people on long term medications would increase, as they would no longer be able to exercise the right not to take them.
- The therapeutic relationship would be damaged, increasing the likelihood of disengagement from mental health services; this could have a particular impact on people from black and minority ethnic groups.
- People, who were not subject to compulsion, might still feel increased coercion in their relationship with services.

---

33 Department of Health (1995), Government Response to the report of the Joint Committee on the draft Mental Health Bill; p.4.
34 Zito Trust; Joint Committee Vol. II, evidence 363.

In general, most critics were not so much concerned about the principle of the use of compulsion in the community, but that it could lead to a substantial increase in the numbers of people who were brought and then kept under compulsion, given that the availability of a hospital bed was no longer a rationing factor. Genevre Richardson described it as a lobster pot – easy to get in but difficult to get out because the broad conditions were very difficult not to meet.[35] The Joint Committee recommended a series of amendments, which would have the effect of narrowing its application to a closely defined group of patients and limiting its scope and potential duration.

Given that one of the pressures for reforming the Mental Health Act was the human rights issues raised by the Bournewood case, it was surprising that the second draft Bill did not address them. A series of measures which appeared in the first draft Bill were removed. These measures extended some of that Bill's safeguards to compliant, incapacitated patients who were detained in hospital, giving them a right to advocacy, the appointment of a nominated person and access to a tribunal. The Government shifted its approach, claiming that safeguards for this group would be provided by the new Capacity Act. This Act provides a statutory framework for decisions about the care and treatment of an incapable person. There does not have to be any formal procedures and no distinction is made between everyday decisions and bigger decisions such as where a person should reside and whether medical treatment should be administered. The proportionate use of restraint is permitted if it is based on a reasonable belief that it is necessary to prevent harm. There are powers to appoint a designated decision maker through the lasting power of attorney provisions or by the appointment of a deputy by the Court of Protection. However, it would not provide sufficient safeguards to cover situations which amount to a deprivation of liberty. As discussed earlier, the European Court of Human Rights held, in the Bournewood Case, that compliance with Article 5 (the right to liberty) would require formalised admission procedures and access to a court to determine the legality of the detention. The Government recognised the need to introduce a new system of 'protective care' where a public authority was involved in arranging a placement for a person who was compliant and incapacitated, where there was deprivation of liberty, so that care and treatment could be provided in the person's best interests.

It is essential that statutory duties and powers, in the area of mental health where questions of individual liberty are involved, are applied fairly and consistently and there are effective safeguards in place to protect against any abuse or misuse of the powers of compulsion. The Government's position was that the Bill "greatly strengthens the safeguards" for patients,[36] notwithstanding that some of the 1983 Act's safeguards have been removed. Nearest Relatives, for example, were to be replaced by the Nominated Person. The patient would have certain rights of nomination, but that Person would no longer have the power to veto an application for compulsory admission or discharge the patient. The Hospital Managers also would no longer have the power to discharge a patient. The Mental Health Act Commission was to be abolished and its functions subsumed under a much larger regularity body, where it

---

35 Professor Genevra Richardson, Joint Committee Vol. II, evidence 11.

36 Department of Health (2004), *Improving Mental Health Law*, Towards a new Mental Health Act, p.7.

was feared that its influence would be marginalised. The Second Opinion Appointed Doctor system would be replaced by an expert panel, which would no longer have the power to veto proposed treatment, which was not in accordance with accepted practice.

The backbone of the Bill's system of safeguards was the requirement that the use of compulsion beyond 28 days must be authorised by an independent judicial body. Stakeholders were generally in favour of the enhanced role for tribunals with the notable exception of the judicial officers of the Mental Health Review Tribunals. They described the new tribunal system as

> unwieldy, unnecessary and unworkable. We believe that the paradigm shift from a reactive to a proactive tribunal has not been thought through at a level of detail necessary to vouchsafe its capacity to achieve what it is intended to achieve, which we understand to be a strengthening of patients' rights to have decisions about liberty assessed with rigour and independence.[37]

They argued that there would be confusion between the judicial function (i.e. the decision about the use of compulsion) and that of a case conference in that the new tribunal would also be required to approve a care plan. They also considered that there would be a conflict between the function of the tribunal as an initial detaining authority and also as a reviewing body when a patient subsequently applied to the same body to review its decision. Their main criticism centred on the resource implications to administer a far larger and more complex system than the current one, which was itself failing to deliver a reliable professional service.

A more fundamental concern raised by other witnesses was the lack of discretion available to the tribunal to discharge patients where the conditions were met. Under the 1983 Act, the tribunal has the power to discharge patients detained under civil powers even though the mandatory grounds for discharge were not satisfied. The discretion might be exercised where the tribunal considered that the medical treatment was not alleviating or preventing a deterioration in the patient's condition or that the patient could otherwise receive the care he or she needed. The Government believed that the conditions allowed the tribunal sufficient flexibility to discharge the patient where compulsion was not appropriate, whereas critics viewed them as being so widely drawn that it would be difficult to see how they could not be met.

There were other safeguards proposed which did find widespread support. There would be a new right to independent mental health advocates. This should be a significant help for patients and the nominated person in ensuring that their views are heard and understood by the care team, provided that there was access to advocacy early enough in the system (i.e. at the examination stage when compulsory powers are being considered) and provided that the service was adequately funded and that its quality and independence were assured. Informal carers were recognised in that there were requirements to consult with them, taking into account the patient's wishes and feelings. The Mental Health Alliance and other critics were also gratified at the Government's change of mind about the omitting of advance directives and statements from the second draft Bill. The Government agreed to include a provision giving an opportunity for patients to record in advance their refusal to receive certain

---

37 Joint Committee Vol. II, evidence 426.

treatments and their treatment preferences. While this would not be binding on clinicians for patients under compulsory powers, they must be taken into account.

The Mental Health Bill was long and complex. Some of the detail has not been discussed in this chapter. For example, no mention has been made of the proposals to restrict the use of ECT, of the special provisions for children and adolescents or patients concerned in criminal proceedings, restricted patients and victims. The Bill was just 23 clauses short of the Lunacy Act, which has been described as a monument to Victorian legalism and was twice as long as the 1983 Act, despite a large chunk having been removed to the Capacity Act. The British Association of Social Workers complained about the "vast amount of obscure, redundant or repetitive verbiage which is quite inappropriate in a statute which has to be operated on a day-to-day basis by non-lawyers."[38] Indeed the complexity of the Bill was such that the Joint Committee made a plea for the Bill to be clearer and easier to read when it was eventually laid before Parliament.

There was still a considerable gap between the Government and its critics even after the concessions made in the Government response to the Joint Committee. Paul Farmer, Chair of the Mental Health Alliance, said,

> After seven years and thousands of hours of consultation on this crucial legislation, some of the basic changes required are now being recognised, but we're a long way from acceptable legislation.

The Government also faced difficulties with regard to the legal obligation under the Race Relations (Amendment) Act 2000 to undertake a race equality impact assessment on the legislative proposals. A group set up by the Department of Health in May 2005 to advise on carrying out such an assessment was critical of the short timescale allowed and the lateness in the legislative reform process in which it was initiated. With the work on the Bill being in its final stages, it was thought that there would be little chance of the race impact assessment resulting in any significant change.[39] The importance of paying attention to race issues was underlined by the first national census on the ethnicity of in-patients in mental health hospitals completed jointly by the Mental Health Act Commission, Healthcare Commission and National Institute for Mental Health in England in 2005.[40] It confirmed the disproportionate use of hospital admission, in particular under the Mental Health Act, for black people.

On 23 March, 2006, the Minister of State for Health, Rosie Winterton, announced the abandonment of a new Mental Health Act. The Government, she said, had taken into account concerns over the length and complexity of the 2004 draft Bill as well as the pressures on parliamentary time, and instead was committed to introducing a shorter, streamlined Bill, which will be easier for clinicians to use and less costly

---

38 Joint Committee Vol. II, evidence 580.

39 Community Care (7 December 2005) News: Bill Faces Legal Threat.

40 Commission for Healthcare Audit and Inspection (2005), *Count me in*, Results of a national census of in-patients in mental health hospitals and facilities in England and Wales. Some of the key findings of this census are summarised in Chapter 2 under the heading of "Visits to Hospitals".

to implement. This Bill would take the form of amendments to the existing 1983 Mental Health Act. There would be six amendments, summarised as follows:

1. To introduce a new, simplified single definition of mental disorder

The Government will keep its proposal from the earlier draft Bill to introduce a single broad definition of mental disorder, so that a diagnostic label will not determine the use of compulsion. The exclusion criteria in the 1983 Act relating to promiscuity, other immoral conduct and sexual deviancy will be removed. However, the Government agreed, in response to some of its critics, to retain explicit reference to dependence on alcohol and drugs as being insufficient on its own, without any other evidence of mental disorder, to justify the use of compulsion. There would also be special provision applying to learning disability, which will keep the limitation of the 1983 Act of only permitting the application of the Act when the disability is associated with abnormally aggressive or seriously irresponsible conduct.

2. To replace the so-called 'treatability test' with a new appropriate treatment test

The clause in the 1983 Act, which only allows compulsory admission in the case of psychopathic disorder or mental impairment, where the treatment is likely to alleviate or prevent a deterioration in the condition, is to be removed. This 'treatability test' has led, according to the Government, to people being labelled untreatable and denied the services that they need. Under the proposed amendment, treatment will have to be available which is appropriate to the patient's mental disorder in all other circumstances. A holistic assessment of the appropriate treatment will be required, which takes account of factors such as distance from, ease of contact with family and friends and cultural needs.

3. To introduce supervised treatment in the community for patients following an initial period of detention and treatment in hospital

Patients already detained in hospital under Sections 3 (admission for treatment) or 37 (hospital order without restrictions) could be made subject to requirements to receive treatment in the community. The responsible clinician, if agreed by the AMHP, will have a power to recall a non-compliant patient to hospital if there are signs of deteriorating mental health. This will be an automatic referral to a tribunal, if the duration of the recall is more than 72 hours.

4. To broaden the group of practitioners who are able to exercise statutory functions

The Approved Social Worker (ASW) is to be replaced by Approved Mental Health Practitioner (AMHP), who could be drawn from nurses and OTs as well as social workers. The local authority will still be responsible for approving AMHPs, but they could be directly employed by health providers.

The Responsible Medical Officer (RMO) is to be replaced by the responsible clinician, drawn from a range of mental health professions trained and approved to take on the role of overviewing the assessment and treatment of the patient. The clinical background would depend on the particular needs of the patient.

5. To strengthen the powers of the Mental Health Review Tribunal (MHRT) as a patient safeguard against long term detention without independent review

This will provide greater protection for patients who do not exercise their right to appeal to the MHRT. Under the 1983 Act, automatic reference by Hospital Managers to an MHRT is made only if a hearing has not taken place in the first six months. Hospital Managers are to be given the power to refer within a shorter timescale. It is intended that these improvements will be made over time and will be dependent on tribunal resources.

6. To remedy a human rights incompatibility and bring the Act into line with the Civil Partnership Act 2004 in relation to Nearest Relative provisions

The Nearest Relative (NR) has been given a reprieve under the proposals to amend the 1983 Act. The government's intention under the original proposals to reform the MHA was to replace the NR with the nominated person with diluted powers. The NR will retain powers to apply for and veto an AMHP's application for detention, discharge the patient, apply to a tribunal and to be given information about the legal status of the patient. However, there will be more flexibility to make an application to the County Court, including by the patient him or herself, to displace the NR. This would cover situations where the involvement of the NR may have adverse consequences for the patient, thereby contravening the human right to privacy and a family life. The displacement could also extend for an indefinite period; i.e. beyond the current episode of admission under the Mental Health Act. For same sex partnerships registered under the Civil Partnership Act 2004, the Act will be recognised with regard to the choice of NR.

In addition to the amendments to the Mental Health Act 1983, it was proposed to make an amendment to the Mental Capacity Act 2005 to introduce safeguards, following the European Court's Bournewood judgment, for people who are compliant, lack capacity and are deprived of their liberty. Hospital and care homes will be required to obtain authorisation from a health or local authority supervisory body if a deprivation of liberty is necessary in the best interests of the person concerned. Such authorisation must be reviewed within a 12 month period. Each person will have someone appointed to represent their interests who is independent of the supervisory body. This may be a family member, a friend or an advocate. There will be a right of appeal to the Court of Protection.

The decision to abandon the 2004 draft Bill was welcomed by many stakeholders, including the Mental Health Alliance. But have the opponents of the Bill shot themselves in the foot? The Government will still be introducing the key contested changes and have abandoned some of the accompanying safeguards.

The definition of mental disorder has been broadened, but there are no proposals to tighten the existing conditions relating to health or safety or the protection of others, as they had intended to do with the 'relevant conditions' listed in Clause 9 of the second draft Bill. It is important that the definition of mental disorder neither excludes those who should be included, nor includes those who should be excluded. There is a risk of the latter if such a broad definition is introduced without extending the limiting provisions to ensure that mental health professionals use their powers in an appropriately narrow way in what has been called the 'broad definition – narrow use' solution. The change in the Approved Social Worker acting as applicant also weakens the consideration of an independent, social perspective. It removes the obstacle of NHS Trusts employing their own Approved Mental Health Practitioners, but then blurs the distinction between the medical decision about the need for treatment and the social decision about whether this should be imposed.

The Government is determined to break the link between the mental disorder and its treatability. This would enable detention to continue indefinitely whether or not the patient is personally gaining any therapeutic benefit as long as he or she is being offered appropriate treatment. In their response to the Government's announcement of plans to amend the Act, the Mental Health Alliance described the proposal for an 'appropriate treatment test' as "too vague and uncertain and therefore not suitable to use when considering the use of coercion."[41]

The Government has kept its commitment to community treatment, albeit limited to patients who have been detained in hospital for treatment in the first instance. There are still concerns that, besides a requirement to take the prescribed medication, a wide range of restrictions could be placed on people living in the community concerning their daily activities. There are fears that patients may be kept under compulsion indefinitely, as there will not be the same pressures to discharge the patient given that the use of compulsion does not depend on the availability of a hospital facility.

The core safeguard of the authorisation by a tribunal of the use of compulsion beyond 28 days has been removed. Although this reform received widespread support, the Government has retreated from its introduction because of potential resource implications. It has also reserved for itself the power to delay implementation of the much more modest reform of reducing the timescale before an automatic review by the Mental Health Review Tribunal takes place.

A right to advocacy was initially not included in the proposed amendments and the Government also back-tracked on its agreement to include advance directives and statements. The patient choice over who takes on the functions of Nearest Relative has also been undermined through the requirement to use the County Court procedure. It will not, for example, prevent an abusive relative becoming involved through his or her right to representation at the Court hearing.

The Bournewood safeguards fall short of those which appeared in the White Paper for Reforming the Mental Health Act and the first draft of the Mental Health Bill and are weaker than those available to patients subject to the Mental Health Act. There is concern that appeals will be heard by the Court of Protection rather that the Mental Health Review Tribunal, which has the necessary expertise in dealing with issues of detention for reasons of mental health. There is also no function for the Mental Health Act Commission or equivalent body to monitor compliance of hospitals, registered homes or the supervisory bodies with the Bournewood procedures.

---

41 www.mentalhealthalliance.org.uk.

The government introduced the Mental Health Bill into the House of Lords in November 2006. There was fierce lobbying and debate, as the Bill yo-yoed between the Houses of Parliament.

The government agreed to a number of concessions, but they gave way as little as possible with regard to the main areas of contention; i.e. the broad definition of mental health, the treatability criteria and compulsory treatment in the community. The government, having already accepted that the single definition for mental disorder would exclude dependence of alcohol and drugs, rejected calls to extend the exclusions to those relating to sexual behaviour or orientation or other immoral conduct. It held on to its position that, as they are not mental disorders, there is no prospect of them being construed as such. It did accept that further guidance about the exclusions is to be given in the Code of Practice. There was a compromise over the 'treatability test'. The Bill was amended to introduce a new 'appropriate medical treatment' test, so that medical treatment for mental disorder shall be construed as applying to treatment where the purpose is to alleviate or prevent a worsening of the disorder or one or more of its symptoms or manifestations. Thus, it is sufficient that the intention of the treatment is therapeutic, whether or not, there is actual therapeutic benefit to the patient. The government strongly defended the community treatment provisions, but agreed to narrow the criteria marginally so that it must be necessary for the responsible clinician to have a power to recall. The proposed wide ranging power that a patient could be made to "abstain from particular conduct" was also dropped.

There were some significant changes in other areas of the legislative proposals, notably in the government finally accepting that advocacy services will be made available for all patients who are liable to be detained or subject to guardianship or a community treatment order. There was considerable wrangling over the role of the Responsible Clinician, which also caused a fracture among the ranks of the Mental Health Alliance. There was a dispute about whether a professional, who is not medically qualified, and acting as a responsible clinician, can provide 'the objective medical expertise', required under Article 5 of the ECHR, to renew detention. It was finally enacted that two professionals from different disciplines will be required to agree renewals of detention. Thus, for the first time, two professionals from different disciplines, neither of whom is necessarily a doctor, will be required to agree renewals for detention. New safeguards were introduced for children under the age of 18, admitted to hospital, so that hospital managers must ensure that the environment is suitable, having regard to the patient's age and needs. Stricter safeguards were introduced over the use of ECT, which can only be given in the face of a capacitous refusal, in an emergency.

The Act received royal assent on 19th July 2007, nine years since the government announced a root and branch review of the Mental Health Act. Some additional matters are, at the time of writing, waiting to be clarified within a Code of Practice, notably the principles which the government refused to include on the face of the Act. The Code is clearly going to be significant in determining how the Act will be carried out in practice. Implementation is not expected until October 2008, at the earliest. So much for a speedy review of the Mental Health Act.

Chapter 5

Socially Determined Perceptions of Risk are Reflected in the Decision to Request a Second Opinion Appointed Doctor's Visit

Hugh Middleton and Ian Shaw

Introduction

A central feature of providing for people with mental health difficulties is the occasional need to consider imposing treatment upon an individual in the absence of their informed consent. Historically patients suffering with mental health problems were considered to lack the necessary judgement or capacity to give true consent. It was not until the 1820s, enlightened by the memoirs of a patient, that awareness of consent became the subject of debate (Perceval, 1982). Furthermore, it was not until the 1970s that the assumption that detained patients could be treated for their mental disorder without consent met serious challenges. The subsequent debate led to the provisions of Part IV of the Mental Health Act 1983, which stipulates safeguards against the inappropriate treatment of non-consenting detained patients. In particular these include the need for treatment plans to be endorsed by a second medical opinion. Current debate and further reform of mental health legislation consider two different sets of circumstances in which treatment without consent might be appropriate. These are either a situation in which a person is considered too psychologically disabled to give fully informed consent (lacks capacity), or circumstances in which a failure to be treated despite lack of consent would put the patient and/or others at risk. Some attempts have been made to clarify how capacity might be determined and assessed. The Law Commission attempted a definition of capacity, which recommends the assessment of five key areas (Law Commission, 1993):

- Communicating a choice – the ability to make a response about a particular decision;
- Understanding information relevant to the treatment – albeit in 'broad terms' and 'simple language';
- Retaining information – if information is not retained, the individual is unlikely to understand relevant information;
- Manipulating information rationally – the ability to weigh the risks and benefits of different options;
- Appreciating the situation and its likely consequences – the individual recognises the disorder for which treatment will apply.

These reflect recent views that the right to self-determination is only meaningful if the person is appropriately informed, is free to make decisions without coercion and has the ability or 'capacity' to make the decision. Where an individual is considered to lack capacity, the individual's need for care and protection from harm supersede considerations of the respect for autonomy (Wong et al., 1999).

Resolution of this tension between respect for autonomy and an individual's need for care routinely relies upon judgements made by medical practitioners and approved social workers. The professional practitioner is primarily responsible for determining whether or not the patient has the capacity to give or withhold consent, and also for defining their 'best interests'.

An important facet of 'best interests' is the notion that psychologically disabled patients can unwittingly be at risk to themselves or to others. Thus, in addition to making judgements about individuals' ability to understand information, consider options and appraise the possible outcomes of treatment, practitioners are also called upon to make a judgement about the extent to which an individual is putting themselves or others at risk. Consideration is given to the possibilities of deliberate self-harm, recklessness, self-neglect, or the extent to which there is risk of violence or dangerousness towards others, or exploitation by them. Thus professional judgements of whether or not a detained patient might be treated against their consent are not only an appraisal of their ability to make an informed decision about the need for treatment but also an appraisal of the risk of self-harm or violence if treatment is not carried out. This could explain why rates of detention deviate from population norms in ways which some suggest reflect a tendency to view certain sections of society as particularly threatening. Noble and Rogers reported a longitudinal record of violent incidents in the Bethlem Royal and Maudsley hospitals in London, and found that, in their control group of non-violent patients, 50 per cent of Afro-Caribbeans in the sample were detained formally on locked wards, whereas only 15 per cent of non-violent White patients were managed in the same way (Noble and Rogers, 1989). Black patients were also recorded as being more violent than White patients. Other investigators of this area have emphasised the need to recognise and respect the effects of cultural distinctions upon the use of services by those of Afro-Caribbean origin (Harrison et al., 1988a).

Such issues underline the importance of considering the relationship between ethnicity and psychiatry, particularly in relation to compulsory admission and treatment without consent. We have used an opportunity to investigate this from the perspective of the Mental Health Act Commission (MHAC) which collects information about patients visited to consider treatment in circumstances where informed consent is not available.

Method

In addition to its visiting programme, the Mental Health Act Commission (MHAC) administers the activities of Second Opinion Appointed Doctors (SOADs). These independent appointees of the Secretary of State review treatment plans for patients in whom the Responsible Medical Officer (RMO) proposes a treatment that requires either consent or a second opinion (Section 58) in circumstances where informed consent is not available, or a treatment that requires both consent and a second opinion (Section 57).

In recent years summary details about patients who have been the subject of such second opinion reviews have been collated by the MHAC as an electronic database. By February 1999 it had accumulated information about 15,466 such visits in the form of 48 variables including: details of ethnicity, gender, age, treatment with ECT and/or medication, Mental Health Act category of illness, whether the patient was deemed incapable of giving consent to treatment or was refusing treatment, section of the Mental Health Act under which detained, and limited geographical information in the form of the Commission Visiting Team catchment area of the visit. We have analysed data from the period March 1997 to February 1999.

The original database was held by the MHAC as an independent mainframe UNIX system. It was exported by tape and reformatted as SPSS, version 8. There was a significant but not disabling rate of missing values (mean rate of missing data per variable 2.5 per cent; range 10.3 per cent (ethnicity) – zero (age and sex)). Extra variables were created classifying ethnicity and age according to the official census categories.

Frequency analysis was used when appropriate, drawing expected frequencies from national statistics of age, gender and ethnicity provided by the Office of National Statistics (ONS) and the Office of Population Census and Surveys (OPCS) (1991 Census).

Results

The database contained information about almost equal numbers of men and women (8,213; 53.1 per cent, 7,234; 46.9 per cent respectively). There were striking differences in the age distribution within each of the genders. Of the male patients, 64.3 per cent were under 40 years of age and 83.7 per cent were under 55. For female patients, 82.7 per cent were over 40 years of age and 62.1 per cent were over 55. Males 17-44 years of age were twice as likely as females of the same age to attract a second opinion visit to consider treatment without consent whereas females 64-85 years of age were twice as likely as males of the same age to attract such a visit.

Table 5.1 gives these age distributions and compares them with those of the general population, defined by the 1991 Census.

Predictably there is considerable under-representation in the 17 and under age group; altogether there were only 277 second opinion visits to persons under the age of 18. Amongst the older age groups there is evidence of over-representation in the 30-44 age range, which was more pronounced amongst men (χ^2 = p<0.001) and amongst females in the over 65s (χ^2 = p<.001).

Understanding Treatment Without Consent

Table 5.1 Gender Distribution by Age Category (per cent Population)

	Gender			
	Male		Female	
Age Category	SOAD Visit	OPCS	SOAD Visit	OPCS
17 and under	1.0	23.8	1.0	20.5
18-29	25.6	19.5	12.9	17.1
30-44	37.7	21.8	24.5	19.9
45-64	21.4	23.3	26.1	21.6
65-74	7.1	8.3	14.8	9.2
75-84	5.8	4.2	14.7	7.5
85 and over	1.5	0.7	6.0	2.1

Figures 5.1 and 5.2 illustrate the ethnic composition of the study population by reference to the 1991 Census. They show, for males and females respectively, the relative difference between the proportion of the population of the second opinion visited patients of a given ethnic background and age band, and the proportion of the general population similarly defined. Later age bands have been omitted because of small numbers: less than 3.5 per cent of the total. These relative differences illustrate the degree to which different age/gender/ethnic background-defined groups of patients were under- or over-represented in the SOAD visit sample. Amongst the males over-representation (Deviation >0) in the 18-29 and 30-44 age ranges is more pronounced amongst those from non-White backgrounds, whereas the converse was true amongst the 45-64 year olds. Amongst the females over-representation in the younger age ranges, though less than amongst the males overall, was also more pronounced amongst patients from Black and Asian backgrounds. Amongst females at the older end of the age range there was over-representation of all ethnic groups.

There were almost equal numbers of visits for issues concerning capacity to give consent as there were for issues concerning refusal to accept treatment, but these had different age and gender distributions which are illustrated in Tables 5.2 and 5.3. Differences between the figures in the latter table and the total numbers of males and females in the sample, 34 males and nine females, are due to missing data.

One thousand, one hundred and seventy-one visits were made to consider the treatment of patients with doses of medication above recommended BNF limits. Males were twice as more likely (797:374) to fall into this category than the gender distribution of the whole sample would predict (χ^2; p<.001). Furthermore there was a significantly higher probability of these considerations applying to patients from minority ethnic groups, which is illustrated in Table 5.3 (χ^2; p<0.001 both genders). Differences between the figures in this table and the overall number of males and females being visited to consider the use of drugs above BNF limits are also attributable to missing data.

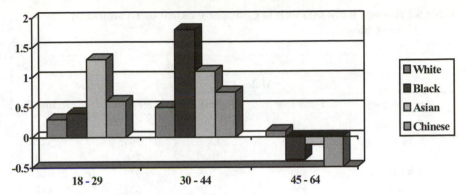

Figure 5.1 Deviation from Parity in the Ratio between the Proportion of the Population of the SOAD Database of a Given Ethnic Background and Age Band and the Proportion of the General Population Similarly Defined: Males

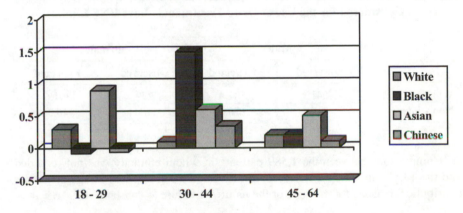

Figure 5.2 Deviation from Parity in the Ratio between the Proportion of the Population of the SOAD Database of a Given Ethnic Background and Age Band and the Proportion of the General Population Similarly Defined: Females

**Table 5.2 Reasons for SOAD Visit to Consider Consent to Treatment by
    Age Category**

Age category	Gender			
	Male		Female	
	Incapable	Refuse	Incapable	Refuse
17 and under	50	28	25	46
18-29	901	1196	394	541
30-44	1265	1809	756	1010
45-64	884	869	923	964
65-74	360	220	638	437
75-84	353	123	721	342
85 and over	99	22	310	118
Total	3912	4267	3767	3458

**Table 5.3 Observed and Expected Frequencies of Whites and Non-Whites
    Considered for the Use of Drug Treatments above BNF Limits**

	Males		Females	
	Observed	Expected	Observed	Expected
White	541	581.4	279	301.6
Non white	217	176.6	63	40.3

Comparisons between the 1,589 patients in whom ethnicity was not recorded and the 13,877 in which it was recorded revealed no differences in age or gender distribution, reasons for the visit, or the nature of failure to consent.

Discussion

These findings are taken from analysis of a robust database. Review of treatment for mental illness without informed consent by a second opinion appointed doctor is a statutory requirement. The source of this information was a database compiled by the body administering those reviews across England and Wales during a two year period and is therefore as good a reflection of the characteristics of patients attracting such visits as can be obtained. Although 10.3 per cent of ethnicity data were missing from the sample, there is no evidence that these missing values were from patients in any way different from the sample as a whole.

The main findings are differing age distributions for patients from the two genders, with a tendency for male patients to fall into the under-45 age range, contrasted with a more even distribution across the age range for females. Compared with population statistics there was significant over-representation amongst male patients attracting an SOAD visit in the 18-44 age range, and amongst female patients in the 65+ age range.

When the ethnic origin of patients attracting an SOAD visit was considered by comparing the ethnic composition of the sample population with population statistics, there was evidence of an over-representation of younger people from the ethnic minorities of both genders. In contrast, the over-representation of elderly females in the sample appears to reflect an over-representation of elderly females from all racial backgrounds.

There is already evidence that people from ethnic minority backgrounds, particularly those born in Britain, are more likely to be diagnosed as suffering Schizophrenia, more likely to be compulsorily admitted to a psychiatric hospital, more likely to be treated in conditions of security and more likely to be given large doses of medication than population statistics would predict (Fennel, 1996). Our findings extend this, confirming the fact that this over-representation includes the use of treatments without consent. Thus, these data are further evidence of an enhanced tendency for young males, particularly those from a minority ethnic background, to find themselves subject to detention under the Mental Health Act and treated without consent than the composition of the general population would predict. Fennel referred to concerns that this might be the case in his earlier report of second opinion visits, and indeed those concerns led to the improved quality of recording ethnicity that this report has been able to take advantage of.

These data also suggest that these over-represented instances of the need to consider treatment without consent amongst younger people are caused by the need to consider circumstances in which a treatment is considered desirable but it is being refused, rather than circumstances in which a treatment is considered desirable and the patient is considered incapable of providing informed consent. A strong inference is that these reflect circumstances in which it is felt desirable to influence patients' behaviour because it is thought to be risky or dangerous, and that inference is perhaps further supported by the finding of an additional tendency to consider the use of neuroleptic medication at doses above recommended limits. Reasons why this might be the case, especially amongst young men from ethnic minority backgrounds are presumably similar to those behind the higher rates of diagnosing Schizophrenia referred to above, and already the subject of a widespread but inconclusive debate around possible explanations. One is that there are higher rates of social disadvantage amongst those from ethnic minority backgrounds. The Fourth National Survey, which measured the socio-economic status of ethnic minorities using three indicators, social class, unemployment rate, and quality of housing, identified the Pakistani and Bangladeshi populations as the most disadvantaged ethnic minority groups (Nazroo, 1997). However these ethnic minority groups do not appear to have rates of mental illness as high as those within the Black population. Although research within this area has produced conflicting results, it is clear that determinants of a high rate of reported psychosis amongst the Black population are more complex than social deprivation alone can explain. Nevertheless Sashidharan strongly discourages dismissing the argument that the relationship between ethnicity and health is a consequence of social disadvantage. Theories suggesting psychiatric disorders to be a consequence of inherent and stable characteristics of certain ethnic minority groups are not only so far untested, but could lead to the cultural and biological heritage of these groups becoming pathologised (Sashidharan, 1993).

Other research has suggested that high rates of Schizophrenia amongst the Black population are the result of stress and other more indirect consequences of social disadvantage (Harrison et al., 1989). As stress and anxiety rates within the Black population appear to be lower than for other ethnic minority groups (Lloyd, 1993), it has also been suggested that high rates of Schizophrenia are related to migration rather than social disadvantage (Sashidharan, 1993). This view is supported by reports of lower rates of Schizophrenia in the West Indies compared to those of the Black population in Britain (Bhugra et al., 1989). This appears to indicate that the process of migration or the way of life upon settlement in Britain affects the rates of Schizophrenia. However, studies have also shown that other ethnic minorities do not have similar rates (Busfield, 1999). Furthermore, the higher rates amongst those born in Britain suggest that there is little to connect the process of migration or straightforward biological or genetic differences to high rates of Schizophrenia. They indicate other factors must be relevant to the increase for the Black population born in Britain. Jenkins states that:

> it is possible, however, that the particular and different ways in which ethnic minority groups are racialised could lead to different outcomes for different groups. (Jenkins et al., 1997)

Furthermore the association between Schizophrenia and violence or other forms of dangerous behaviour links violence and dangerous behaviour not only to Black males within mental health in general but also specifically within the population of patients who are detained and, in particular, do not comply to consent to treatment (Cope, 1989). Some suggest that a diagnosis of Schizophrenia automatically labels the patient as dangerous or violent, especially in those cases involving males from amongst the Black population (Boyle, 1990).

This draws attention to the need to acknowledge the way in which culture determines rates of illness and raises the question of how much of a particular diagnosis is based on perceptions of illness, characteristics of the individual patient or misunderstandings about minority cultures.

Cultural dimensions of illness within Western bio-medicine, or what has been called the 'category fallacy' (Kleinman, 1980), have lead to cross-cultural comparisons of mental health. This amounts to:

> the reification of a nosological category developed for a particular cultural group that is then applied to members of another culture for whom it lacks coherence and its validity has not been established. (Mirowsky and Ross, 1989)

The judgement of whether behaviours and actions are symptomatic of abnormal mental health requires, he argues, knowledge of their social and cultural context. Within psychiatry, the definition of disease and dysfunction is often very unclear.

> Cultural factors play a far more significant role in the recognition of mental disorders than they do in physical illness. What may be considered as a departure from normative

behaviour in one culture may not have the same meaning when applied to another culture. (Bentall, 1988)

We have presented data from a robust source that clearly illustrates an un-representative tendency to use statutory powers that enable treatment without consent upon young males and, to a degree, young males and females from ethnic minority backgrounds. A brief review of possible explanations for an over-representation of persons from ethnic minority backgrounds amongst those detained under the Mental Health Act suggests that simple factors such as an inheritable propensity, or a direct association with social disadvantage, or 'stress' do not provide an adequate explanation. That it is not just individuals from ethnic minorities that are over-represented amongst those being considered for treatment without consent but, just as strikingly, young males of all races suggests that it is more likely that this over-representation reflects real or perceived risks of violence occurring in the context of what might be construed as mental illness.

There are culturally bound determinants of the response to different forms of dangerousness and these inevitably influence professional judgements. Pilgrim and Rogers suggest that "professionals have an interest in maintaining a construct which in common cultural currency equates mental illness with violence" (Pilgrim and Rogers, 1999). They also argue that this common perception, that the mentally ill are more aggressive, is driven by the media. The influence of the media in shaping views about violence and mental disorder has increasingly been a cause of great concern. Philo reported that two-thirds of items dealing with mental health issues forged a link with mental illness and violence (Philo et al., 1994). These judgements are also influenced by a public perception of the young black male as a more dangerous person. It is the male Afro-Caribbean community, fuelled by the media publicity of particular incidents, which is more likely to be linked with crime and violence (Ritchie et al., 1994).

That this ethnic bias appears to be reflected in rates of detention under powers of the Mental Health Act and rates of treatment without consent suggests that practitioners administering Mental Health Act procedures are themselves not immune to these public perceptions; indeed it has long been argued that maintaining a social order based upon shared perception is part of their legitimate role (Porter, 1987). Similarly, O'Malley has argued that the welfare state is changing its role in response to the development of a risk society (O'Malley, 1991) whereby the role of the State is to protect citizens against risks perceived as unpredictable. It would seem that the behaviour of certain subgroups of individuals deemed to be dangerous by virtue of mental illness falls into this category.

References

Bentall, R.P., Jackson, H.F. and Pilgrim, D. (1988), 'Abandoning the concept of schizophrenia: some implications of validity arguments for psychological research into psychotic phenomena', *British Journal of Psychology*, 27, 303-324.

Bhugra, D., Hilwig, M., Hossein, B., Marceau, H., Neehall, J., Leff, J., Mallett, R. and Der, G. (1996), 'First contact incidence rates of schizophrenia in Trinidad and one year follow-up', *British Journal of Psychiatry*, 169, 587-592.

Boyle, M. (1990), *Schizophrenia: A Scientific Delusion*, Routledge: London.

Busfield, J. (1999), 'Mental Health Policy: Making gender and ethnicity visible', *Policy and Politics*, 27, 57-73.

Cope, R. (1989), 'The compulsory detention of African-Caribbeans under the Mental Health Act', *New Community*, 15, 343-356.

Fennel, P. (1996), *Treatment without Consent. Law, Psychiatry and the Treatment of Mentally Disordered People since 1845*, Routledge: London.

Harrison, G., Holton, A., Neilson, D., Owens, D., Boot, D. and Cooper, J. (1989), 'Severe mental disorder in Afro-Caribbean patients: some social, demographic and service factors', *Psychological Medicine*, 19, 683-696.

Harrison, G., Owens, D., Holton, A., Neilson, D. and Boot, D. (1988), 'A prospective study of severe mental disorder in Afro-Caribbean patients', *Psychological Medicine*, 18, 643-657.

Jenkins, R., Lewis, G., Bebbington, P., Brugha, T., Farrel, M., Gill, B. and Meltzer, H. (1997), 'The National Psychiatric Morbidity Surveys of Great Britain: Initial findings from the household survey', *Psychological Medicine*, 27, 775-789.

Kleinman, A. (1980), *Patients and Healers in the Context of Culture*, University of California Press: Berkeley.

Law Commission (1993) 'Mentally Incapacitated Adults and Decision-Making: Medical Treatment and Research' Consultation Paper No. 129.

Lloyd, K. (1993), 'Depression and Anxiety among Afro-Caribbean general practice attenders in Britain', *International Journal of Social Psychiatry*, 39, 1-9.

Mirowsky, J. and Ross, C. (1989), 'Psychiatric diagnosis as reified measurement', *Journal of Health and Social Behaviour*, 30, 11-25.

Nazroo, J.Y. (1997), *Ethnicity and Mental Health: Findings from a national Community Survey*, Policy Studies Institute: London.

Noble, P. and Rodger, A. (1989), 'Violence by psychiatric in-patients', *British Journal of Psychiatry*, 53, 384-390.

O'Malley, P. (1991), 'Legal networks and domestic security', *Studies in Law, Politics & Society*, 11, 181-191.

Perceval, J. (1982), 'A narrative of the treatment experienced by a gentleman during a state of mental derangement', in D. Peterson (ed.) *A Mad People's History of Madness*, pp.106-107, University of Pittsburgh Press: Pittsburgh, PA.

Pilgrim, D. and Rogers, A. (1999), 'Mental Health Policy and the Politics of Mental Health: A three tier analytical framework', *Policy and Politics*, 27, 13-24.

Porter, R. (1987), *Mind Forged Manacles: A History of Madness in England from the Restoration to the Regency*, Athlone: London.

Ritchie, J. et al. (1994), 'The impact of the mass media on public images of mental illness: media content and audience belief', *Health Education Journal*, 53, 271-282.

Sashidharan, S.P. (1993), Afro-Caribbeans and schizophrenia: the ethnic vulnerability hypothesis re-examined, *International Review of Psychiatry*, 5, 129-143.

Wong, J.G., Clare, I.C., Gunn, M.J. and Holland, A.J. (1999), 'Capacity to make health care decisions: Its importance in clinical practice', *Psychological Medicine*, 29, 437-446.

Chapter 6

To Treat or Not to Treat?
Should the Treatability Criterion for
Those with Psychopathic Disorder
be Abandoned?

Conor Duggan

Abstract

The detention of an individual with Psychopathic Disorder in hospital under the 1983 Mental Health Act is unique in requiring that the condition be 'treatable'. Although this criterion was introduced to protect the patient from unlawful detention, many believe that it had the paradoxical consequence of excluding individuals from care that might otherwise benefit them. As a result, psychopathic disorder has been excluded entirely in the revision of the Mental Health Act.

Nonetheless, the provision of treatment is of central concern when any mentally disordered individual is detained against his/her will. This chapter will consider the necessity of treatment and its various interpretations for those with psychopathic disorder (with or without a history of sexual offending) with reference to two landmark Court rulings (i.e. Kansas vs Hendricks, 1997; and ex parte A, 1995). History shows that this criterion of treatability is a mixed blessing for those with psychopathic disorder, having both unfortunate consequences as well as the intended benefits. The recent service development to incarcerate those with severe personality disorder who are deemed to be dangerous (i.e. DSPD), and where treatability is no longer a criterion of entry, alarms many professionals who see this as a means of preventative detention without the checks and balances of the previous system. Despite difficulties in both its definition and implementation, therefore, I will argue that it is the anchoring of decision making within accepted clinical norms that provides the best protection for the patient and clinician alike, when decisions on the detention of personality disordered individuals are required to be made.

Introduction

Psychiatry is unique as a medical sub-specialty in being able to detain and treat an individual in the absence of his/her consent based not on the individual's lack of capacity, as would apply in other medical disorders, but rather on certain features associated with mental disorder itself. The general conditions allowing this to occur within the England and Wales 1983 Mental Health Act are that (a) the individual being detained suffers from the disorder in question and (b) that this places him/her at risk of harm either to self or others. In the case of psychopathic disorder, there is an additional requirement that the condition is 'treatable'. It is this third criterion of treatability and its consequences that is the focus of this chapter.

There are some obvious questions to consider. Why, for instance, is the criterion of 'treatability' restricted to psychopathic disorder and not applied to other mental disorders? What does it mean and how is it applied in practice? Is the proposed abandonment of psychopathic disorder a good or bad development in the proposed new mental health legislation? Many of these questions take on a particular resonance with the development of specific services for those who are deemed to be dangerous and have a severe personality disorder (the so-called DSPD services). Here, entry to the service is dependent on the presence of the following triad: (a) severe personality disorder, (b) dangerousness and (c) a 'functional link' between (a) and (b). While each of these criteria will be subject to challenge, I suspect that it is the 'functional link' that will be the most contentious criterion. Nowhere, however, is it stated that the individual has to be 'treatable'.

Although it is only in the case of Psychopathic Disorder that treatability is explicitly necessary to justify detention, a focus on treatability is implicit in the practice of psychiatry for all mental disorders when individuals are being detained. The argument advanced is that, while there has been a loss of liberty for the individual (i.e. hospitalisation for most detained patients has been seen as essentially a form of imprisonment), this is justified (in the professionals' minds at least) as there is an assumed benefit for the patient from being so detained. This principle of reciprocity (i.e. the patient gives up his/her freedom, albeit involuntarily, in the expectation that some form of effective treatment will be offered in return) is the key feature that distinguishes involuntary incarceration from punishment in the criminal justice system. Paul Applebaum (1988), for instance, contrasts the respective state of prisoners as compared with mental health patients in the following terms:

> Unlike prisoners in a pure preventative detention system, patients committed to mental health facilities receive direct benefits from their detention beyond those in society at large might derive ...

Providing treatment for the psychiatric condition then is clearly *the* important condition that ought to be met when one is depriving anyone of their liberty for this purpose. This general 'principle of reciprocity' ought then to underpin all involuntary incarceration in mental health services. But what does this mean in practice? As the line between detaining for treatment or imposing preventative detention is one that is easily crossed, Applebaum (1988) went on to specify three criteria that need to be met so as to prevent the misuse of psychiatry for this purpose. According to Applebaum, detaining an individual for treatment requires it be limited to (a) those patients who are treatable in the setting to which they are sent, (b) the actual provision of the said treatment, and (c) detaining individuals only as long as to accomplish the needed treatments. While these criteria appear almost as 'psychiatric givens', they lead to important implications.

For instance, it follows from (a) and (b) that the clinician has to be satisfied, not only that the patient is 'treatable' but also by implication that the treatment is effective and that he/she is in a position to deliver the treatment. Thus, airily stating that the patient's condition is in principle 'treatable' is insufficient for detention according to these criteria unless one has the means to deliver the effective treatment. It is further implied in (c) that the individual ought to be detained only as long as it is necessary to deliver the proposed treatment, irrespective of the risk that he/she might pose in other respects at the completion of treatment. This might typically arise when a convicted criminal at high risk of re-offending is transferred from prison to hospital because he/she has become psychotic. Applebaum makes it clear that, once the psychosis has been resolved, the individual either should be returned to prison to complete his/her sentence or be released to the community if they have passed their release date while being treated in hospital and that this should occur irrespective of the risk that they might pose on release.

All three criteria ought to cause clinicians to pause and think. First, they pre-suppose that there is evidence for the effectiveness of the intervention. I shall argue later that the evidence for many treatments for psychiatric conditions is weak, in some cases indeed to be almost non-existent, so that many would not be able to withstand this challenge. The recent focus on practice that is evidence based together with the development of NICE Guidelines, Cochrane Reviews etc. are all likely to place the effectiveness of the treatment of any disorder (mental disorders included) increasingly in the spotlight (Klerman, 1990). Second, is it legitimate to detain someone compulsorily for a treatment if that treatment cannot be provided? This would arise when a specific therapy for a condition is required but, say, the funds for that treatment or the personnel to deliver it are not available. The individual is potentially treatable but the means are not there to offer the appropriate treatment. Applebaum makes it clear that such an individual ought not to be detained. This illustrates the dyadic nature of treatability so that it does not reside solely in the individual being treated but in the broader system in which he/she is a part.

Kansas vs Hendricks (1997)

Nine years after Applebaum set out his criteria, some of its implications were tested by the US Supreme Court in Kansas vs Hendricks (US Supreme Court Reports, 1997). The background to this case is worth stating as, although it refers to the preventative detention of those who are likely to re-offend sexually, it shares many features with the proposed DSPD development. Briefly, in 1994, the State of Kansas enacted a Sexually Violent Predator Act that allowed the civil commitment (i.e. the preventative detention) of persons who, due to their 'mental abnormality' or 'personality disorder' are likely to engage in 'predatory acts of sexual violence'. Thus, if an individual had (a) a previous history of sexual violence and a mental abnormality and (b) was judged to be at high risk of further re-offending, then it was justifiable to preventively detain him.

Shortly after the legislation was enacted, a convicted paedophile (Leroy Hendricks), soon to be released from prison having served a fixed-term sentence, was deemed to be of such high risk of re-offending that, just before his release, he was committed to a further period of indefinite detention in order to prevent him doing so. Hendricks challenged his continued committal and was successful initially in the Lower Kansas Court, only for the decision to be reversed by the Kansas Supreme Court. The case was then referred to the US Supreme Court.

After considering the evidence, the US Supreme Court found in favour of the Kansas Supreme Court (i.e. that civil commitment was lawful) on a split 5/4 verdict. Two considerations stand out from the Chief Justices' deliberations that are relevant for our purpose. The first of these is that they were satisfied that a broad definition of 'mental abnormality' or 'personality disorder' was satisfactory. This is somewhat surprising in view of many mental health professionals that personality disorder diagnosis in particular has unacceptable temporal and convergent reliability (Zimmerman, 1994). Hence, although there is poor inter-rater agreement both when the assessments are repeated over time or when different assessments are compared one with another, the Court was satisfied that this broad description of the mental disorder (i.e. 'personality disorder') was acceptable.

More importantly for our purposes, however, was how seriously the Chief Justices took the necessity of treatment in such cases. They referred, for instance, to the Allen vs Illinois (1986) decision, in which it was stated that "... the State has a statutory obligation to provide 'care' and treatment for persons (adjudged sexually dangerous) designed to effect recovery ..." Further, in a telling phrase from the same case, treatment was described as "... a kind of touchstone helping to distinguish civil from punitive purposes."

Echoing the earlier requirement from Applebaum (1988), the importance of the practical delivery of treatment was highlighted by Justice Kennedy – clearly one of the wavering Justices – when he wrote "If the object or purpose of the Kansas law had been to provide treatment but the treatment provisions were adopted as a sham, or mere pretext, there would have been an indication of the forbidden purpose to punish" (US Supreme Court's Reports, 1997).

In summary, the US Supreme Court added the necessity of treatment to the Kansas Supreme Court's earlier criteria allowing preventative detention. Hence, in future, the formula for preventative detention would read – a history of a relevant offence, the presence of a mental disorder and the likelihood of a repetition of the earlier offence and the provision of treatment – as the necessary criteria enabling the State to detain an individual preventatively.

Looked at superficially, it would appear that this addition of treatment was an important condition as it provided the individual with something while at the same time denying him his liberty. Its provision after all was "... deigned to effect recovery" and hence must be a good thing. Looked at another way, however, does not the availability of treatment enable preventative detention to occur in the first place? If, for instance, there was no treatment available, would this mean that the individual could not be preventatively detained? Treatment therefore has a Janus-like quality – both for good or ill – depending on which way the face is turned.

R vs Cannons Park Mental Health Review Tribunal

To my knowledge, we have no similar clarifying legislation on 'treatability' in the UK comparable to that of Kansas vs Hendricks in the US. Nonetheless, there is one case which addresses these issues – albeit in a more limited form – that I will now consider. This is R vs Cannons Park Mental Health Review Tribunal. It has already been discussed usefully in an article by Baker and Crighton (1995) "Ex parte A: psychopathy, treatability and the law", from which this is a distillation.

This case involved whether the treatability criterion for Psychopathic Disorder under the 1983 Mental Health Act (viz. that medical treatment in hospital "... is likely to alleviate or prevent a deterioration of the patient's condition") was properly met. (Due to the controversial nature of Psychopathic Disorder, the criterion of treatability was introduced in the 1983 Mental Health Act as an added protection for the patient against illegal detention.)

The background to this case was as follows. A (the patient) had a history of depression, deliberate self-harm and alcohol dependency and was detained under Section 3 of the 1983 Act under the legal designation of mental illness. Subsequently, her Responsible Medical Officer (RMO) changed the legal categorisation by which she was detained to that of Psychopathic Disorder. In so doing, he made it clear that the 'treatability test' was satisfied. In this case, the 'treatment' consisted of psychotherapy offered in a group setting.

Subsequently, A made it clear that (a) since she was unwilling to comply with group treatment, (b) it meant that she was 'untreatable' and (c) she ought therefore to be released. On this basis, she appealed against her continued detention under the 1983 Act to the Cannons Park Mental Health Tribunal. Despite her arguments and the Mental Health Tribunal acceptance that this medical treatment was unlikely 'to either alleviate or prevent a deterioration in her condition' as A refused to comply, it nevertheless refused A's application to be discharged.

A then applied for a judicial review to the High Court. At this review, Justice Sedley found in her favour stating that "... it was never appropriate under the provisions of the 1983 Act ... for a patient to be detained in a hospital for medical treatment for psychopathic disorder if he or she is not at that point treatable."

Cannons Park MHRT then appealed the Sedley decision to the Court of Appeal and the latter reversed the previous decision finding in favour of the MHRT – again on a split 2:1 verdict. One of the Judges (Justice Kennedy) argued that

> ... there was evidence before the tribunal ... that over a prolonged period of treatment, consisting at first of not more than nursing care and persuasion to accept group therapy, followed by group therapy itself was likely to prevent deterioration of her condition, even if at first some deterioration could not be avoided ... that this might eventually lead to an improvement in the patient's condition.

This definition of treatment, a definition that is reiterated later in the Justices' judgment, gives those who provide the treatment an extraordinary degree of latitude. It implies, for instance, that initially treatment in hospital (defined as no more than "... nursing and includes care, habitation and rehabilitation under medical supervision") is sufficient to fulfil the criterion of treatability. Hence, for the Judges at the Court of Appeal, simply being detained in hospital is sufficient in itself as a form of treatment although this enforced hospitalisation was exactly the point that was before the Court for a decision.

Although the Judges make explicit the purpose of such a hospitalisation – namely that the patient gets insight into his(/her) condition so as to "… cease to be un-co-operative in his attitude toward treatment which would potentially have a lasting benefit", this decision, while being appealing, raises as many questions as it seeks to answer. First, is this not a subtle way of coercing an individual into treatment? Although coercing someone into treatment is a complex issue whose implications need to be thought about carefully, nonetheless for those with personality disorder whose compliance with any treatment regime is almost a sine qua non of developing a therapeutic alliance, this form of compulsion raises significant issues of therapeutic engagement.

Second, the Justices were clearly anxious to avoid a situation where the patient was able to dictate their treatment from the beginning and thereby determine their release. In fact, the Appeal Court acknowledged this in the case of A for, if she were granted release on the basis of her non-compliance (i.e. being deemed untreatable), this would set a precedent for other detained patients to also achieve their release by not complying. The Appeal Judges clearly saw the unacceptable implications of this, concluding that "Were this to be accepted, patients would deem themselves untreatable simply by withholding their co-operation. That would place the key to the patient being detained in hospital in the patient's own hands which would not have been Parliament's intention."

Those who participate in Mental Health Tribunals on patients in high security hospitals detained under Psychopathic Disorder will be well aware of patients refusing to participate in any further treatment, lest this be interpreted as an acknowledgement of the need for yet more treatment in a high secure hospital. Here, the patient is in a 'Catch 22' situation; if he/she admits the need for further treatment, then he/she will continue to be detained until this is accomplished. If, however, he/she denies the need for such treatment, this is interpreted as 'a lack of insight' that requires further treatment in a high secure hospital until this is effected. On the surface, at least, the patient is dammed whatever he/she does; this clearly is unacceptable.

There were two conclusions from the ex parte A case. The first was that the different criteria of treatability were to be applied to patients entering hospital from those leaving it. The second is that the treatability criterion could now be defined very broadly indeed; so broadly that it is difficult to know how it might afford any patient protection against wrongful detention. This asymmetrical application of the treatability criterion to those outside hospital compared to those within it led one commentator to conclude dryly that the "… new treatability test is designed to protect the hospitals from any responsibility towards patients whom they do not want, but provides no protection at all for the patient who does not want the hospital" (Hoggett, 1990).

Currently, therefore, there is an uneasy standoff between clinicians on the one side and patients on the other. Clinicians, for the most part, wish to avoid caring for those with personality disorder as they believe they (a) have little to offer them but more importantly (b) wish to avoid the responsibility when such patients misbehave

– especially violently. The patients comprise two groups: (a) an increasing number of disgruntled individuals in secure facilities wishing to end their treatment and (b) a much larger group in the community who wish to obtain it (NIMHE, 2003). Surely, we can do better than this.

A Way Forward?

I would argue that three conditions are necessary if this area is to advance. First, we need to apply better and more precise definitions of the disorder and clarify the purpose of treatment. Second, we need to make it clear that, while those with personality disorder have rights to treatment, this has to be accompanied by them accepting responsibility for their behaviour. This applies particularly to those with personality disorder who commit offences. Third, we need to identify the causal connections between the disorder and the offences. This will be no mean undertaking but will be important as it will probably identify a very small number where there is a connection and who require specialised help and that these need to be separated from the very large number of offenders who coincidentally also suffer from personality disorder. Fourth, we will need to be able to produce evidence that effective treatments are available. None of these are undertakings but it is important that we make a beginning. Let me therefore expand briefly on what I mean.

(a) Problems of Definition

It is crucial that we clarify our definitions of personality disorder as failure to do so will perpetuate the problems of the past when very vague definitions can become over-inclusive. This is both unfair to an individual who might inadvertently get caught up in such a system and a major problem for research as the inclusion of non-cases as cases add 'noise' to the system. A typical example is the legal term 'Psychopathic Disorder' as this contains a very heterogeneous group, including many with a diagnosis of mental illness (Blackburn, 1992). One of the objections to accepting one of the current diagnostic systems for personality disorder is that they have many deficiencies so that, by accepting them, we are perpetuating one error with another. While one accepts that current diagnostic systems are inadequate, at least they are a beginning and what objectors do not seem to realise is that the most rapid way of demonstrating the deficiencies in a system is to have clear definitions so that it can be put to an empirical test.

An example may help to make this clear. There is a belief that very psychopathic individuals do badly with treatment (Rice et al., 1992). This has led to a policy decision within the prison system to deny very psychopathic individuals access to many psychological programmes in custodial settings as it is believed that these would harm the inmate. For those being deprived of treatment, this is a very important decision that could affect their release. However, is this policy justified?

Clearly, it would be impossible to answer this question unless one had a universally agreed definition of what constituted a very psychopathic individual. Such a definition exists, namely a high score on the Psychopathy Checklist – Revised

(PCL-R) (Hare, 1991). In fact, there is evidence that someone who scores in the 75th percentile or above in North America or in the 63rd percentile or above in the UK is prone to both increased recidivism and a poor response to treatment. Hence, these are the data that influenced the Home Office in its selection of inmates for prison treatment programmes.

D'Silva et al. (2004) carried out a systematic evaluation of whether the evidence from the literature justified official policy. They found that, because of serious methodological inadequacies in the few studies that had addressed this question, one was unable to answer this question either way. They concluded that it is not so much that this policy decision is wrong as that it is premature.

I am discussing this at some length, not to criticise the Home Office – although I do believe that they have made a decision on inadequate evidence – rather, it is to say that this review could not have been carried out to any purpose if the authors were unable to anchor their investigation to generally accepted definitions of psychopathy. Hence, such narrow but clear definitions encourage refutation as well as confirmation, thereby allowing knowledge to advance.

In this respect, I welcome use of explicit entry criteria to the proposed DSPD services. Therefore, for someone to gain entry to the service, he (and it is restricted to men at the moment) must satisfy all of the following triad: (a) have a severe personality disorder, the definition of which is anchored to clearly defined criteria (i.e. the presence of DSM or PCL-R criteria that are quite explicit), (b) meet criteria of dangerousness that again use accepted instruments to define it and (c) show a 'functional link' between (a) and (b). While one might disagree with the assessments and the definitions provided, it will nonetheless now be possible to have a debate on them in a way that was not possible in the past. Additionally, if these are properly applied, this will provide some protection for the patient.

(b) Rights and Responsibilities

This is an area that mental health services generally try to avoid and I believe do so to their disadvantage. Putting niceties of definitions aside, I believe that there are some 'psychopaths' who either through temperamental or characterological abnormalities (and I believe that temperament is the more salient) lack a moral compass so that their interaction with others is severely compromised. Richards (1998) describes such individuals as rarely experiencing normal guilt and self-esteem. He goes on

> Mens rea, guilty intent, does not exist on the subjective level for such individuals. Instead, pathological identifications and renunciations, both at the unconscious level of object relations and at the conscious level of belief systems and values, engender intentions centered on aggression and destructiveness. This evil intent, or ill will, becomes essential to the individual's self-cohesion.

Richards' point is that such individuals have a limited capacity (or perhaps no capacity) to choose life over destructiveness.

If that is the case, and if this is dependent as much on biological underpinnings as Richards' early identifications, what effect ought this to have on judgements of guilt? Surely, these individuals – and they are a tiny, though important minority – cannot be held responsible for their actions as they clearly lack 'guilty intent' as they are incapable of experiencing 'guilt'. In what sense then, are such individuals responsible for their actions and how should they be punished when they transgress the law (Blair et al. 1995)?

If the absence of guilt in such cases is used to excuse the behaviour, what about the borderline personality disordered individual who makes rash choices with adverse consequences to others because he is unable to weigh up the cost of a choice (however high) when faced with a substantial reward? And what about antisocial adults who have a sense of entitlement that excuses their misdeeds because of the deprivations they have suffered in the past? Clearly, the extension of mental disorder to explain (and excuse) criminal behaviour, parodied beautifully by Officer Krumkie in West Side Story, will not be tolerated by society.

Not only is society unwilling to accept an infinite extension, personality dis-ordered individuals themselves ought to reject it for the following reason. For, is it not the case that disavowing responsibility for one's behaviour in this way suggests such a lack of self control that control by the State becomes necessary? Murphy (1972), for instance, concludes that because psychopaths are outside the realm of obligation they therefore have no moral rights. The cost of disavowing responsibility for one's behaviour therefore is extraordinarily high and this indeed is the position in which a few unfortunate individuals in high secure care find themselves. Although they (and their advocates) may have convinced the judicial system that they are incapable of being responsible for their actions and therefore have gone to hospital, they need to be aware that they will subsequently have to convince clinicians of the reverse in order to get out. This is a much easier exercise for those with mental illness as it is good evidence that medication is effective in at least reducing the symptoms of the illness and therefore of reducing the risk (assuming the risk is related to the presence of the illness). The position is more difficult for those with a personality disorder or psychopathy where the evidence of treatment efficacy is much less compelling.

Here again, treatability is a consideration. Clinicians have been criticised (sometimes fairly) in refusing to offer treatment to those with personality disorder, especially in secure settings. When this decision is seen in the rights vs responsibility debate, however, this refusal might be to the patient's advantage for, if the treatment is offered and it turns out to be unsuccessful so that effectively the individual is consigned to incarceration for a very long time, has it done the patient any favours?

Surely the most pragmatic position to adopt at the present time is, first, for patients with personality disorder to accept that they are responsible for their actions, even though in many such cases the presence of the disorder may reduce the level of responsibility (and in a very small number of extreme psychopaths perhaps eliminate it completely); for to do other would open them to indefinite incarceration. Second, accept that treatment can be offered to those with personality disorder but only to those who are sufficiently responsible to accept it voluntarily. Hence, a personality disordered individual who is convicted of a crime ought to face the same consequence as would anyone else. Subsequently should he/she wish to have treatment, this request is treated as would any similar request and offered if it were deemed appropriate. Hence, the most pragmatic way of moving forward is to accept that those with a personality disorder are as responsible as anyone else for their actions (criminal or otherwise) and they are also as entitled to the same rights to treatment as anyone else. Acceptance of this position would free mental health professionals from having to provide treatment to those who either (a) do not want it and (b) are unable to benefit from it.

(c) A Causal Link between the Disorder and Offending

It is important to consider this as it is one of the entry criteria to the DSPD services. Here, the individual must (a) not only have a severe personality disorder and (b) be dangerous, but there has to be a causal connection between (a) and (b). This is an important issue when we come to discuss the outcome from treatment (qv. below); it assumes that if one eliminates or reduces the severity of (a) with treatment then the offending (or 'dangerousness') will also be reduced as a result.

Unfortunately, for the proponents of this argument, the data supporting this causal connection are either non-existent or contradictory. For instance, Bonta, Law and Hansen (1998) conducted a large meta analysis to identify the antecedents of re-offending among mentally disordered offenders. They found that the predictors of re-offending among this group were the same as in offenders without a mental disorder (i.e. being male, young, unemployed etc.) so that the mental disorder per se accounted little for variance in the re-offending behaviour. Although, among all the mental disorders, personality disorder was the only one that showed a positive association, this cannot be used as strong evidence as (a) the association was weak and (b) there is significant overlap between the diagnosis of antisocial personality disorder and criminality.

This approach can be rebutted as it is too molar and therefore lacks the precision required to find an association. The argument is that a more detailed examination of specific personality disorders and specific types of offending is required if an association is to be found. Here again, unfortunately, the empirical data are almost non-existent as the author has only been able to find a single empirical study that is relevant. This is a study by Coid (1998) who examined the types of offences committed by those with a range of personality disorders who were detained either in High Secure Hospitals or Special Prison Units. In general he found that the proposed association between the specific personality disorders and specific types of offending to be weak (i.e. his Confidence Limits were very large). Putting this objection to one side, together with the methodological flaw that the investigator was not blind to the offence when the personality disorders were rated, there is a more serious objection to using this type of exploratory analysis to justify the identification of a causal link. This is that no causal mechanism was proposed connecting the personality disorder to the specific form of offending. Consider, for instance, Coid's most impressive finding that borderline personality disorder (BPD) was related to the offence of arson. Unfortunately, this association does not take us very far as BPD in DSM is a heterogeneous condition involving abnormalities in affect, identity and impulsivity. In order to have a testable theory, one ought to identify the particular traits within BPD that are associated with arson. If, for instance, it is hypothesised that it is impulsivity that leads to fire setting, then an intervention that reduced impulsivity ought to have the consequence of reducing arson. Unfortunately, personality disorder research currently lacks this type of theory (Epstein, 1988).

(d) Effective Treatments for Personality Disorder

In the light of the deficiencies in (a) and (c) above, it is no surprise that identifying effective treatment for personality disorders has lagged behind those that tackle more symptomatic presentations of mental disorder (e.g. such as the reduction of psychotic symptoms). With personality disorder, however, the ground rules for treatment are much less clear. What exactly is the outcome in the treatment of personality disorder? Is it a fundamental change in personality structure (whatever that might mean)? Is it a reduction in some behavioural manifestations such as re-offending in the case of ASPD or deliberate self-harm in those with a borderline diagnosis etc? Mental Health professionals here neatly avoid considering such fundamental questions as to (a) whether personality (disorder) changes and (b) if it does, then what is the evidence that it does so (Duggan, 2003)? Yet, without agreement on such a fundamental question, it is difficult to see how the area will advance.

Putting aside the difficulty in deciding on an outcome measure in personality disorder, the issue of whether or not there is evidence to justify intervening in any personality disorder remains. We have recently completed a systematic review on the efficacy of psychological and pharmacological interventions for personality disorder and have found that high quality evidence justifying the interventions is very poor generally and is almost non-existent for antisocial personality disorder. In that condition, for instance, we could find only three studies that satisfied the Cochrane standards for entry into a systematic review (Duggan et al., 2005).

In the high stakes involved (e.g. detaining someone without limit of time until treatment has effected a change) and the disagreement among professionals, it is surprising that this absence of evidence receives so little comment. For instance, if a child had a serious blood disorder that required an immediate transfusion but its Jehovah's Witness parents were against such an intervention, I believe it would be possible to go to a court and seek to do so with good evidence that such an intervention would save the child's life. It is difficult to believe that a similar case could be made to a Court when detaining someone for treatment for an indefinite period of time. The science of the discipline will clearly have to progress significantly for this to occur.

Conclusion

Given the difficulties of the current position, it is easy to understand why the Government (and some members of the profession) would wish to abandon treatability as a criterion for the access to service provision for those with personality disorder. Within the proposed new Mental Health Act, for instance, there is no separation of the different types of mental disorders so that mental illness, learning disability and psychopathic disorder are all grouped together under the generic term 'mental disorder'. Again, within the new Act, the disorder has to be of a nature and degree to require treatment, that this treatment is necessary for the protection of the patient and others and, finally, that appropriate treatment 'be available' for the person's disorder.

While it is clear that drafting legislation of this type has to be general, it is unclear if this will in any way avoid the mistakes and controversies of the past. In order to do so, what will be required is more science, rather than less. I believe that it is only when there is evidence that personality could be diagnosed reliably and validly, that treatments are available that clinicians agree have an acceptable evidence base, that individuals were free to access them if and when they choose; then and only then, will the patient be properly protected. A change in the law in itself will I suspect achieve little, unless it is accompanied by a major advance in scientific knowledge.

References

Applebaum, P.S. (1988), 'The New Preventative Detention: Psychiatry's Problematic Responsibility for the Control of Violence', *American Journal of Psychiatry*, 145, 779-785.

Baker, E. and Crichton, J. (1995), '*Ex parte* A: psychopathy, treatability and the law', *Journal of Forensic Psychiatry*, 6, 101-109.

Blackburn, R. (1986), 'Patterns of personality deviation among violent offenders: replication and extension of an empirical taxonomy', *British Journal of Criminology*, 26, 254-269.

Blair, R.J., Jones, L., Clark, F. and Smith, M. (1995), 'Is the psychopath "morally insane"?', *Personality and Individual Differences*, 19(5), 741-752.

Bonta, J., Law, M. and Hansen, K. (1998), 'Prediction of criminal and violent recidivism among mentally disordered offenders: A Meta-Analysis', *Psychological Bulletin*, 123-142.

Coid, J. (1998), 'Axis 11 disorders and motivation for serious criminal behaviour', in A. Skodol (ed.), *Psychopathy and Violent Crime*, pp.53-97, American Psychiatric Association: Washington, DC.

D'Silva, K., Duggan, C. and McCarthy, L. (2004), 'Does treatment really make psychopaths worse? A review of the evidence', *Journal of Personality Disorders*, 18(2), 163-177.

Duggan, C. (2004), 'Does Personality Change and, if so, what changes?' *Criminal Behaviour and Mental Health*, 14, 5-16.

Duggan, C., Adams, C., McCarthy, L., Fenton, M., Lee, T., Binkes, C. and Stocker, C. (2005), 'A Systematic Review of the Effectiveness of Pharmacological and Psychological Treatments for those with Personality Disorders', *Report for the National Forensic R & D Programme*.

Epstein, S. (1987), 'The relative value of theoretical and empirical approaches for establishing a psychological diagnostic system', *Journal of Personality Disorders* 1, 100-109.

Hare, R.D. (1991), *The Hare Psychopathy Checklist-Revised*, Multi-Health Systems, Toronto.

Hoggett, B. (1990), 'Mental Health Law', 3rd edition, Sweet & Maxwell: London.

Kansas vs Hendricks (1997), US Supreme Court Reports Nos. 95-1649 & 95-9075.

Klerman, G. (1990), 'The psychiatric patient's right to effective treatment: Implications of Osheroff vs Chestnut Lodge', *American Journal of Psychiatry*, 147, 409-418.

Murphy, J.G. (1972), 'Moral death: A Kantian essay on psychopathy', *Ethics,* 82, 284-294.

Rice, M.E., Harris, G.T. and Cormier, C.A. (1992), 'An evaluation of a maximum security therapeutic community for psychopaths and other mentally disordered offenders', *Law and Human Behaviour*, 16, 399-412.

Richards, H. (1998) 'Evil Intent: Violence and Disorders of Will', in T. Millon, E. Simonsen, M. Birket-Smith and R.D. Davis (eds.), pp.69-94, *Psychopathy: anti-social, criminal and violent behaviour*, Guilford Press: New York.

Zimmerman, M., (1994), 'Diagnosing personality disorders: A review of issues and research models', *Archives of General Psychiatry*, 51, 225-245.

Chapter 7

Law, Regulation and the Mental Health Act Commission

Simon Boyes and Michael J. Gunn

Mental Health: Regulating Risk

Regulation, whatever its form, is traditionally associated with the prevention of harm or the risk of harm. Law and regulation of mental health does not differ from this norm. Historically, it is clear that legal regulation of mental health provision has been premised upon concerns for public safety. The extent to which these concerns were material appears uncertain in retrospect. Nevertheless, it is clear that initial drivers for regulation in this area were founded deeply in public concern over the management and control of the 'insane'.

The permissive approach to incarceration established by the Vagrancy Act 1744, in particular the role of the judiciary rather than the medical profession in making determinations regarding admissions to asylums, is illustrative. Far from being an issue of treatment, the regulation of mental health at this early stage seemed to be focused on the management of the perceived effects of mental illness. This is entirely consistent with the key rationale for regulation.

Broadly conceived, regulation takes place where the overall environment – embracing the legal, political, economic and societal elements – fails to deliver outcomes deemed appropriate in the prevailing social climate (Francis, 1993). Allowing the insane to remain 'at large' gave rise to the perceived possibility that they would pose a threat to the wider public. This is a reason *par excellence* for the imposition of a regulatory strategy.

> [R]egulation exists because in its absence, as historical record demonstrates, the result is the wide scale production of death, injury and illness, destruction and despoliation, not to mention systematic cheating, lying and stealing. (Tombs, 2002)

While this may appear extreme, Tombs identifies the key rationale of regulation: the prevention of harm. What emerges through consideration of the legal regulation of mental health is that developments in such regulation have largely been driven by shifts in the perception of harm and the nature of the overarching politico-legal environment. Earlier chapters in this collection highlight the rationale for the early law in this area as being motivated by concerns over high profile homicides perpetrated by 'lunatics'. Similarly, the drive towards greater accountability and individual justice during this early period seems to have been fuelled by public concern about the operation and practices of institutions. Such an approach is not uncommon in regulatory terms. The more 'rustic' early approach to mental health regulation focused primarily on the physical harm which could be inflicted upon members of the public by the mentally ill. The incarceration and physical restraint of patients, while addressing the underlying concern pertaining to the harm which they may cause to others, brought about a shift in regulatory focus towards potential harm brought about by the control activity itself (see, for example, the discussion of Lomax in Chapter 2 of this book).

This is well illustrated by the development of the role of the Lunacy Commission. It developed from an oversight body, with investigative and informational functions, to a rule approver under the 1853 Act with the introduction of more stringent legal mechanisms under the 1890 Act. Nevertheless, the legalism engaged under the 1890 Act remained focused upon the primary aim of mental health regulation during that period – protection of the general public from the 'dangerous' mentally ill. Legal safeguards were concerned very much with insuring against 'inappropriate' release of inmates from incarceration. This is not incongruous with a period in British history in which the prevailing political drive was towards control and prevention of disorder – a period of 'civilization' (Elias, 1981). Codification and development of rules and regulations was fashionable during this time. For example, the codification of the criminal law pertaining to non-fatal bodily harm, the Offences against the Person Act 1861, still applies today. It should come as no surprise therefore that these two trends produced the societally-focused outcome represented by mental health regulation. It is, perhaps, equally unsurprising that regulation in this area has struggled to free itself from the shackles of its early form. This is not untypical in any field of regulation. Early approaches often dominate the area for many years thereafter, even when it becomes apparent that such an approach is inappropriate for modern times. Conservative approaches, to change from the regulated and the regulator, can often result in a degree of 'regulatory lag' occurring (Hancher and Moran, 1998); there is clear evidence of this in the field of mental health regulation, with the death of the then Earl of Shaftesbury clearing the way for a new approach under the Lunacy Act 1890 (highlighted in Chapter 2 of this book).

Nevertheless, the conservatism inherent in regulatory structures can still be thrown off. This much is evident from the shift in regulatory strategy after the Second World War. The shift towards communitarianism in the immediate aftermath of war, particularly in the field of health with the introduction of the National Health Service, had a clear impact upon the regulation of mental health. This move in the field of health generally was compounded by a broader societal shift towards the protection of individual rights as a political priority. The conclusion, during this period, of a raft of global treaties on human rights and in Europe the creation of the Council of Europe and the attendant European Convention on Human Rights, in which the United Kingdom was at the forefront, provided a vastly different political culture in which mental health regulation operated. Similarly, revulsion at the atrocities committed against the mentally ill in Nazi Germany provided a more specific impetus for regulatory reform (Eastman, 1994).

Despite this, it was not until the reforms of the Mental Health (Amendment) Act 1982, their consolidation into the Mental Health Act 1983 and the consequent creation of the Mental Health Act Commission (MHAC) that regulation in this area shifted focus substantially towards the protection of the patient from its skewed position as being solely concerned with the protection of the public, despite the presence of public concern from the late 1800s. Nevertheless, as noted in Chapter 2 of this book, this regulation has been the subject of fierce criticism in the restriction of its scope solely to those detained under the Act.

There is one other motivator in mental healthcare that must be recognised, and this is paternalism. Whilst the key principle, in general, for healthcare is respect for the principle of autonomy (so that capacitous individuals make their own decisions), there is a very clear tradition for acting for another's benefit when that other has a mental illness (or other mental health problem). The Mental Health Act 1983 allows for this, since admission can be compulsorily imposed either because others need protection from harm or because the intended patient's health or safety requires it. Such a driver seems to have currency both in the general population and in the relevant healthcare professions, as can be seen in the relative lack of objection to maintaining a paternalistic justification for compulsory detention in the reform of the Mental Health Act 1983.

The Mental Health Act Commission: Regulatory Role

Approaches to legal regulation of any area of concern inevitably require a 'regulator'. In many cases regulation by the 'ordinary' law of the land, civil and criminal, is sufficient. However, where special situations arise which fall without this generic spectrum, specialist bodies are often preferable. In the context of the regulation of mental health, there has been preponderance towards what has become known as 'decentered' regulation (Black, 2001). Under this approach the regulation of the activity is undertaken by a body designated specifically for the task, which is, at least to a degree, independent of the State. Where regulation is carried out by the State direct, in this case the Department of Health (and its precursors), this can often result in 'over regulation'. Such models tend towards complexity and inflexibility. Indeed, for these and other reasons, the management of the special hospitals has been removed from the Department and placed within the NHS Trust structures that operate in the Health Service generally. The 'command and control' model often meets with hostility from the regulated industry. It can have difficulty obtaining important information, upon which it will base its regulatory strategy, from the regulatees. Also, rigid structures (whether by the State itself or other regulatory bodies) tend to lead to legal defensiveness and a lack of cooperation from the regulated sector. Indeed, the initial draft of the Mental Health Act Code of Practice met with vociferous resistance from both the Royal College of Psychiatry and the British Medical Association, largely due to what was perceived as its over-prescriptive nature.

Considered from the State perspective, moving regulation of a particular area away from the centre has manifold benefits, many of which are particularly apt in the context of mental health. In a complex area such as this it is likely that effective regulation will demand a high level of relevant expertise on the part of the regulator; such knowledge and understanding will not only make it easier for the regulator to make well informed choices, but also enhance perceived legitimacy amongst the regulated group (Baldwin and Cave, 1999). Further, those with an intimate knowledge of the regulated sector are likely to enjoy easier access to the information required to set rules and standards and more readily to understand that information and its consequences. This reduces costs. More importantly, it enables the regulator to enjoy a greater degree of trust on the part of the regulated group. In addition, creating specialist bodies with attendant detailed knowledge makes decision making quicker and, importantly for governments, cheaper. Indeed, the relatively light-touch regulatory approach manifest in the MHAC seems largely to be a result of a desire to promote a partnership between the regulator and the regulated sector. However, regulatory relationships of this type often give rise to accusations of regulatory 'capture'. This means that the overseeing body is subject to undue influence from the sector and begins to act in a way which favours the industry rather than following its specific remit (Baldwin and Cave, 1999). Bodies such as the MHAC are ripe for capture in this way. Since it has no powers of compulsion, it is reliant on the goodwill of the industry for the implementation of policy. Even where a body has enforcement powers, capture by the regulated body, or parts of it, is still a recognised risk. As a body, the MHAC seems almost primed for capture. In its creation and membership, the Commission can be perceived as a 'carve up'; the result of a bargaining process between those groups with relevant interests in this area. The form of the regulator and, indeed, the substance of regulation itself can often be the result of competing interest groups both within and outside the sector itself. In the context of mental health, it is possible to perceive a clear tension between a variety of concerns, as noted in Chapter 2. Jones identifies these as the medical, legal and social interests. This tension was manifest from the early days of mental health regulation, with the 'splitting' of the Lunacy Commission between the legal and medical professions. This, it seems, is a trend which has carried on, as the MHAC has continued to be dominated by these professions in the ensuing years. The nature of the regulator and the 'shape' of regulation itself is ultimately determined by the extent to which different interest groups occupy 'regulatory space' (Baldwin and Cave, 1999; Francis, 1993). The result is usually the adoption of a compromise position. Inevitably, the State is a key player in this process. The extent to which the State chooses, is compelled or is able to involve itself in the regulation of a sector is highly significant in shaping regulatory space. This is not least because the State is usually representative of society's underlying political and legal philosophy. This is evidenced by the significant conflict, between the MHAC, Department of Health and professional bodies representing the various sectors of the medical profession, in drawing up the original MHA Code of Practice (Cavadino, 1995).

The use of codes of practice forms a significant part of 'de-centred' regulation. Codes are described as 'quasi-legislation'. They provide an opportunity not only for the application of specialist knowledge in a particular area but also for a degree of 'buck passing' by governments and legislators (Cavadino, 1993). Indeed the function of developing the Mental Health Act Code of Practice assigned to the MHAC has been perceived by some as the organs of State 'ducking' difficult issues in the face of vociferous and polar views from a variety of interest groups (Cavadino, 1993).

Despite this, perhaps cynical, view it is widely accepted that disputes are resolved much better by a specialist body familiar with sectoral issues than by a generalist body which must appraise itself of these on each occasion which it is called upon to adjudicate. Indeed, the Mental Health Act Commission has been able to gain a high degree of compliance within the sector, despite the absence of any 'hardcore' regulatory tools at its disposal and attendant allegations of 'toothlessness'.

> The MHAC, while a well respected and competent body, is hampered by the fact that it is remote; commissioners can only visit establishments caring for seconded patients once or twice a year. It lacks any power to compel provider units to follow good practice and can only 'name and shame' in its biennial reports. It cannot review complaints unless they have not been satisfactorily settled by hospital managers. It has no power to discharge patients from section, nor does it concern itself with the treatment of voluntary patients. (Gregory, 2000)

As considered elsewhere in this work, the Mental Health Act Commission has a number of statutory responsibilities allocated to it, with an overall responsibility to act as 'watchdog' in respect of those compulsorily detained under the MHA 1983. The MHAC has a brief to maintain a review of the MHA 1983, visit and interview patients detained under the Act, the investigation of complaints relating to the treatment of detained persons, the appointment of psychiatrists authorised to give second opinions pertaining to compulsory treatment under the Act and the development and maintenance of a code of practice to supplement the Act (MHA 1983, ss. 120 and 121). Essentially, the function of the MHAC is the oversight of the period of detention. The Commission has no role in determining whether or not to detain patients, or in decisions pertaining to their release. This function is reserved for the courts and Mental Health Review Tribunals. The latter have the power, in relation to all detained patients, to order their discharge (except those transferred from a prison sentence, whom it can order to be returned to prison) and patients have periodic rights of application. The Tribunal, therefore, has the power to determine whether to continue the detention of a detained patient. Given the level of interference with the liberty of an individual, the quasi-judicialisation of this process appears entirely appropriate. The removal of an individual's liberty is a serious prima facie infringement of their human rights and as such both domestic law and the European Convention of Human Rights demand that such action is both justifiable and determined in an appropriate fashion. Nevertheless, the remit of the MHAC is of considerable importance. It is the only body with a regulatory responsibility for the position of a patient once detained, at which time many freedoms are consequentially affected. There are consequences that flow as explicitly provided for in the legislation, most importantly when treatment can be provided, in many cases without the consent of the patient (Mental Health Act 1983, Part IV), but also including, e.g. limitations upon correspondence (Mental Health Act 1983, s. 134). Further, there are implicit consequences that flow from being a detained patient as first identified in Pountney vs Griffiths ([1976] AC 314, HL) in relation to the ability to use force to escort someone between ward and visiting areas. Subsequently, it has been recognised that the consequences can include such matters as the use of seclusion (see, e.g., R (Munjaz) vs Mersey Care NHS Trust [2003] EWCA Civ 1036), and the use of telephones (R (N) vs Ashworth Special Hospital Authority [2001] HRLR 46). Since the focus of the Commission is on the in-hospital period, its remit is of considerable importance. It has, indeed, taken on board the checking of compliance with Part IV, at least through checking the compilation of the forms authorising treatment under sections 57 and 58. Further the Commission has the remit to examine the use and practice of seclusion, by endeavouring to secure compliance with the Code (see the Munjaz litigation).

Assessing Regulation: The Mental Health Act Commission

The Scope of Regulation

Perhaps the most significant criticism which can be levelled at the Mental Health Act Commission is that of overt and excessive paternalism in respect of the approach to treatment of patients detained under the MHA 1983. Whilst its remit in relation to patients in hospital is of considerable significance, the MHAC has only limited powers to review the treatment of individual patients. It lacks any kind of authority to award remedies to those aggrieved. In contrast to the highly individualised nature of the detention/release decision making process, the role of the Commission is much more concerned with a broader oversight of the treatment of detained patients. Section 120(1)(b)(ii) MHA 1983 allows the Commission to investigate complaints about "all those rights and duties which flow necessarily and by implication from a Section 3 detention … such rights and duties as necessarily flow from the Act" (R vs Mental Health Act Commission, ex parte Smith [1998] 43 BMLR 174). This is a welcome expansion of what the MHAC itself had previously believed to be a much more limited role (MHAC, 1999). But, it also has the power to "keep under review the exercise of the powers and the discharge of the duties conferred or imposed by this Act so far as relating to the detention of patients or to patients liable to be so detained …" (section 120(1), MHA 1983). It is this power that enables the Commission to have oversight of both the explicit and implicit powers that flow from detention (indeed in relation to correspondence there is a specific role as in s. 134; and there are specific roles in relation to oversight of Part IV on consent to treatment, though its remit clearly runs further than such specific roles). Focus on this remit is of high importance. Whether the Commission has operated this function sufficiently effectively is open to doubt. In any case, it is significant that the approach to admission/release remains more closely regulated. This reflects a regulatory culture where the focus is on the protection of the public at large from the 'dangerous' mentally ill and, to a degree, protection of the patient themselves. The enforced detention of patients has been the subject of significant judicial scrutiny, and has developed accordingly. In contrast, there appears to be little consideration of the necessary infringement of liberty incurred when an individual is made subject to treatment. To a degree, it appears the case that an automatic presumption of incapacity arises when an individual is detained compulsorily.

Limited Remedies and Regulatory Capture

On complaint investigation, whilst R vs Mental Health Act Commission, ex parte Smith represented a welcome expansion of the capacity of the MHAC to consider the treatment of detained patients, it remains the case that the Commission retains the discretion to decline to investigate, or indeed to terminate any investigation. In any case, the MHAC may only investigate complaints where hospital management has been unable to satisfactorily resolve matters, effectively obscuring the regulator's view of many problems within the system. Further, it has not consistently exercised its broad function under section 120(1) as effectively as it could have done. Whilst the forms authorising treatment under sections 57 and 58 were usually read on a visit to a hospital, it is not clear that problems were readily identified or referred to the hospitals, nor is it readily apparent that the significance of this work was truly recognised. In any case, the MHAC is necessarily impaired by its lack of remedial powers. Its most effective power is, in its report to a particular hospital or trust, to raise specific issues that demand attention and then to follow those up. This presumes that it has the capacity to identify and follow up effectively. Clearly, its ability to do this improved over the years, but it is very dependent upon the effectiveness of a part time group of Commissioners and their understanding of the key agendas of the Commission. Further, the MHAC having the power to 'name and shame' in its published biennial reports presented to Parliament is useful. Not only may it provide guidance to mental health professionals and institutions, but also no public body relishes such public ignominy. Nevertheless, the measure is severely limited in its ability to provide justice for detained individuals. All of this means that there is the potential for one of two polar situations to arise. First, that the MHAC becomes so reliant on the goodwill of mental healthcare providers that it is effectively 'captured', limited to regulating with the 'approval' of the regulated. In the alternative, it may be that the MHAC as a regulator is largely ignored by the sector, given the limited remedies available to it. Addressing these matters would require a full time Commission, as in Scotland, that had a clear agenda in relation to reviews of "the exercise of the powers and the discharge of the duties conferred or imposed by the" Mental Health Act 1983 (MHA 1983, s. 120(1)). It would have to have clear enforcement powers, such as the right to refer a case to a Mental Health Review Tribunal or to a lawyer for consideration of taking legal action or to the Health Service Ombudsman.

Conclusions

All of the above demonstrates that, while the MHAC has achieved much in promoting good practice in relation to the treatment of detained patients, there remain concerns that the body is not sufficiently 'heavyweight' to give appropriate redress and protection to an exceedingly vulnerable group. These anxieties are unlikely, it seems, to be redressed by any new mental health legislation, which looks increasingly likely to see an end to the MHAC. The protracted period of consultation and political horse-trading which has so far taken place suggests that the most probable outcome will be the abolition of the MHAC and the dispersal of its powers and responsibilities between the burgeoning group of regulators in mainstream healthcare (McHale, 2003). Such a development, without any attendant enhancement of associated powers, is likely to be a retrograde step. The MHAC has, for the most part, been able to make the most of its limited authority; much of this can be ascribed to the specialist knowledge and focus of the Commission. These advantages will, more than likely, be diluted with the scattering of the Commission's functions. Not only this, but under the MHA 1983 the MHAC deals with a peculiar niche in healthcare regulation; because of the acute interference in individual liberty necessarily involved with involuntarily detained patients, the Commission deals with difficult issues that a more generalist healthcare regulator may not have the knowledge, expertise or specialist understanding of. Consequently, individual civil liberties may suffer.

References

Baldwin, R. and Cave, M. (1999), *Understanding Regulation: Theory, Strategy and Practice*, OUP: Oxford.

Black, J. (2001), 'Decentering Regulation: Understanding the Role of Regulation and Self-Regulation in a "Post-Regulatory" World', *Current Legal Problems*, 54, 103.

Cavadino, M. (1993), 'Commissions and Codes: A Case Study in Law and Public Administration', *Public Law*, 333.

Cavadino, M. (1995), 'Quasi-government: the case of the Mental Health Act Commission', *International Journal of Public Sector Management*, 8(7), 56.

Eastman, N. (1994), 'Mental Health Law: Civil Liberties and the Principle of Reciprocity', *British Medical Journal*, 308, 43.

Elias, N. (1981), *The Civilising Process*, Blackwell: Oxford.

Feintuck, M. (2004), *The Public Interest in Regulation*, OUP: Oxford.

Gregory, P. (2000), 'Who can best protect patients' rights', *Psychiatric Bulletin*, 24, 366.

Hancher, L. and Moran, M. (1998), 'Organising Regulatory Space' in R. Baldwin, C. Scott and C. Hood, (eds.), p.148, *A Reader on Regulation*, Blackwell: Oxford.

McHale, J. (2003), 'Standards, quality and accountability – the NHS and mental health: a case for joined up thinking?', *Journal of Social Welfare and Family Law*, 25(4), 369.

Mental Health Act Commission (1999), *The Mental Health Act Commission: Eighth Biennial Report 1997-1999* (London, The Stationery Office).

Tombs, S. (2002), 'Understanding Regulation?', *Social and Legal Studies*, 11, 113.

Chapter 8

Reforming the Mental Health Act: A Successor to the Mental Health Act Commission

Jeffrey Cohen

In 1998, the Department of Health announced that there would be a 'root and branch review' of the Mental Health Act. It established the Mental Health Legislation Review Team (the Richardson Committee) to "advise on how the mental health legislation should be shaped to reflect contemporary patterns of care within a framework which balances the need to protect the rights of individual patients and the need to ensure public safety" (DoH, 1999[1]). The proposition that the Mental Health Act Commission (MHAC) or equivalent specialist body would have a key role within the new legislative framework was rarely questioned during the early stages of the review. There was a consensus that being made subject to compulsory intervention, for reasons of mental disorder, requires additional safeguards and oversight from a body constituted for the purpose. Paul Boateng, then Minister of State for Health, in his opening remarks to the Richardson Committee specifically asked it to consider how the current MHAC functions might be revised so that any successor body "can address the whole issue of service quality whether for detained or informal patients."

The reference to informal patients is significant. There is provision in the 1983 Mental Health Act for the MHAC to look into matters relating to informal patients, but only when directed by the Secretary of State. Such a direction has not been given, despite repeated MHAC requests for an extension of its remit to cover de facto detained patients. Here, for the first time, there was an indication of ministerial approval for such an extension. This change in the Government's position had been prompted by the Bournewood case,[2] which highlighted the gap in safeguards for the compliant, incapacitated patient, whose status was that of informal patient. Another gap in the MHAC's remit has been the lack of any oversight over the use of compulsion in the community in the form of Guardianship or Supervised Discharge. Although not explicitly stated in the introductory remarks of the minister, given the governmental imperative that compulsory treatment would not be tied to detention

---

1   Department of Health (1999), Report of the Expert Committee: Review of the Mental Health Act.
2   R vs Bournewood Community and Mental Health Trust ext parte L [1998] 3 AER.

in hospital, the remit of the successor body would necessarily apply to patients under compulsion whether in hospital or community settings.

In an unpublished paper prepared by the Sainsbury Centre for Mental Health in 1999,[3] the option of abolishing the MHAC and distributing any continuing functions to other regulatory bodies was considered, but was not regarded as practically or politically feasible. There would, it was thought, be a possibility, or probability, of a severe loss of focus on the rights and quality of care of detained patients when the work becomes a small part of other agencies' responsibilities. It was suggested in the Sainsbury Centre paper, that any disadvantage could be reduced by making the functions into a distinct sub-office of an existing organisation. But, again, it was thought that the loss of a single identifiable agency would lead to severe criticisms from stakeholders and there would be high political cost. Three years later, support for the MHAC had declined to the extent that the political risk of abolition did not appear so great and the Government put forward the model of incorporating the monitoring functions within a division of a new health care inspectorate, the Commission for Health Audit and Inspection (known as the Healthcare Commission).

A wider remit for the Commission had also been mooted by the House of Commons Health Committee. It recommended that "the role, powers and resources of the Mental Health Act Commission should be reviewed with a view to their extension to cover all designated mental health services." It also proposed that it should have representation on the national level of other regulatory bodies.[4]

Submissions to the Richardson Committee confirmed the support for an extension of the role of the MHAC in new legislation. The Committee envisaged that the new body would be an "important additional safeguard for patients in its role as a guardian of the interests of individual patients" with its primary focus being towards individual care and treatment. It also recommended that, while the primary duty would be towards those subject to compulsion, its responsibilities should extend to informal patients. Besides monitoring the treatment and care of those subject to compulsion whether in hospital or community and monitoring compliance with the legislation and code of Practice, the Richardson Committee outlined a number of other key functions. Notably, it recommended that the successor body should become a repository of knowledge and information about the legislation. It should receive notification of all uses of compulsion and have responsibility to monitor, analyse and publish such data in a Biennial Report to Parliament. It should have the power to provide legal practice advice about the implementation of compulsory powers and have some involvement in the provision or accreditation of training for those with responsibilities under the Act. It was recommended that it should also be given a new power to refer a patient's case to a tribunal. The complaints remit of the current Commission should not continue, but it should have a general power to investigate any matter which falls within its jurisdiction and it should still receive

---

3   The Sainsbury Centre for Mental Health (1999), *The Functions and Structure of the Successor Body to the Mental Health Act Commission*, unpublished.

4   House of Commons Health Committee (1999), *Fifth Report on The Regulation of Private and Other Independent Healthcare*, The Stationery Office.

reports of all those patients who die while under compulsion and have the power to investigate the circumstances. It should also be able to identify themes for scrutiny.

The Richardson Committee recommended that the new body be fully independent of State agencies and of Government and be answerable directly to Parliament, possibly through the Health Select Committee.

The DoH, in the Green Paper[5] which followed the Richardson Committee's report, did not commit itself to what shape the MHAC successor body might take, but indicated that it should be formed in the context of other measures to improve the quality of health and social services. It emphasised the importance of not duplicating the functions of other regulatory bodies, but should complement them through additional safeguards for patients subject to compulsory powers.

In response to the Green Paper, the MHAC issued a special paper "A Successor to the MHAC",[6] in which it put forward a strong argument for a separate body, to safeguard the interests of those subject to compulsion, which is independent from the NHS and lead governmental department. "Coercive powers," it was argued, "imposed by the state for therapeutic reasons can be misused, even if for benevolent reasons. The general public needs to be reassured that all reasonable steps have been taken to prevent this and also, more generally, to be confident that mental health legislation cannot be used for social engineering or political purposes." Further justification for an independent body was that none of the new health related bodies have a remit exclusively related to the effects of compulsion on patients. These bodies are also more concerned with general standards and quality of service delivery than with particular individuals. Later in the paper, it was suggested that there would be cost and management advantages in the successor body having a role in the administration of the Mental Health Tribunal service. "Using the same databases of people," it was argued, "for the successor body's dedicated functions and for the Tribunal could avoid unnecessary duplication, conflict of interests in individual cases, and confusion of roles." The Sainsbury Centre had considered this option and concluded that, while it would create economies of scale, it would be unlikely to attract much support. Significant practical and legal conflicts could arise and the priorities could become distorted with a bias towards legal rather than quality aspects of the role (The Sainsbury Centre for Mental Health, op cit).

The MHAC went on to identify five key functions which the successor body should have; namely visiting, monitoring, reviewing (including complaints and deaths), reporting and dissemination, and acting as a focus for other bodies with an interest in mentally disordered patients.

The *visiting* function was regarded as essential, as there can be no real safeguard for individuals that does not involve personal contact. It is necessary to ensure that patients have been informed of their rights under mental health legislation, are receiving appropriate care and treatment, are not being subjected to unnecessary or improper use of restrictive powers (e.g. seclusion, control and restraint, refusal of

---

5   Department of Health (1999), Reform of the Mental Health Act 1983. Proposals for Consultation. Cm 4480. London DoH.

6   MHAC (2000), A Successor to the Mental Health Act Commission. Response to the Green Paper Reform of the Mental Health Act. MHAC, Nottingham.

leave or visits or access to activities) and know how to make a complaint if they are dissatisfied with any aspect of their care and treatment. Interestingly, there was no mention of visiting in the Green Paper, although, at this stage, it was not apparent that the Department of Health intended to remove this function.

Visiting is also necessary for *monitoring* purposes, so that an independent check can be made with compliance on the ground with the formal requirements of the legislation and Code of Practice. The monitoring role of the MHAC has been limited by the lack of statistical data on uses of the Mental Health Act. One of the extensions of the functions of the successor body could be a statutory right to receive notification of all admissions/changes to and discharges from compulsory powers. This statistical information would point to general trends and variations in the application of the Act between individual units. When combined with qualitative analysis of findings from visits, such information would enable local differences to be analysed and pointers to good or bad practice identified.

The MHAC's response to the Green Paper envisaged that the monitoring of information collected on visits and through statistical analysis would be reinforced by a *reviewing* function which would enable "the successor body to satisfy itself that the spirit as well as the letter of the relevant legislation was being implemented." The MHAC has carried out a number of thematic reviews of matters of particular importance to the operation of the Mental Health Act through questionnaires administered on each visit or through a National Visit, in which a sample of units was visited on the same day. The Richardson Committee explicitly recommended that the successor body should have the power to identify specific themes for scrutiny.

The MHAC advocated a significant expansion in its successor body's activities relating to the *reporting and dissemination of information*. Findings from visits and statistical analysis and guidance on the operation and interpretation of mental health and related legislation could be published in a variety of formats, including the statutory report to Parliament, annual reports and other publications. The body could provide an advice service, including maintaining a web site, on legal and practice issues and changes in mental health case law. It could also have a role in training for practitioners with responsibilities under the Mental Health Act.

The Richardson Committee saw the MHAC successor body as being a main player at national level in maintaining standards in mental healthcare generally. It recommended that the successor body should "create working links with all relevant regulatory and other similar bodies and to provide a *focus* for all agencies and bodies involved in the provision of mental healthcare." The MHAC itself was more circumspect in its response to the Green Paper. Despite previous exhortations for its remit to cover informal patients, who are de facto detained, the MHAC strangely no longer favoured the inclusion of informal patients within its statutory remit. It was thought that this would detract from the focus on compulsion, which is the main justification for a separate body. More general matters of treatment and care, the MHAC maintained, are the concerns of management and other national bodies with responsibilities for monitoring the quality of service delivery.

The White Paper "Reforming the Mental Health Act" was published in December 2000 and announced that there would be a Commission for Mental Health, fully independent of the NHS. It specified that the remit would, in fact, extend to covering the care of patients with long term incapacity, who were not formally detained. It would be given new responsibilities for collecting and analysing information and overseeing standards of specialist advocacy and training for practitioners operating the Mental Health Act. However, the new Commission would not have responsibilities for regular visiting. The visiting function was to be taken over by the Healthcare Commission or the Commission for Care Standards. The specialist advocacy service would take over the role of alerting patients to their rights and responding to issues raised by patients. The Commission for Mental Health would be responsible for assuring the quality of specialist advocacy services and providing advice and support to advocates.

The Commission was still expected to keep the operation of the Act under review and to advise the Secretary of State whether the powers in the Act are being used appropriately. While mental health commissioners would be able to accompany or advise the other Commissions on inspection visits, without a dedicated visiting function, it is hard to envisage how the Commission for Mental Health would be in close enough contact with the day-to-day operation of the Act and the concerns of patients to keep the Act under review or maintain credibility in its ability to do so.

To all intents and purposes, the White Paper scuppered the proposals that the MHAC had put forward for the future of its successor body. The visiting function was abandoned and the White Paper made no mention of the Commission for Mental Health providing a focus for other agencies in mental health. Without the visiting function, the monitoring and reviewing functions would be weakened. The Commission for Mental Health would not, on its own accord, be able to identify themes for scrutiny or carry out reviews on matters of particular importance. Of the five main functions identified by the MHAC, only that of reporting and disseminating of information remained intact.

The structure and functions of the successor body were to be diluted even further at the next stage in the reform of the Mental Health Act, the publication of the first draft Bill in July 2002. Alongside this draft, the Government issued a consultation document, seeking further views on various matters, including the scrutiny functions to be included in the future Bill. No mention was made of a Commission for Mental Health. Instead, it was proposed that the role of scrutinising the proper application of the new Mental Health Act would be carried out by a specially established division of a new health care inspectorate, the Commission for Health Audit and Inspection (Healthcare Commission) with the following functions:

- collecting information;
- investigating/visiting for cause: this would supplement the role of the specialist advocacy service by giving an additional power to visit patients where there is cause for concern about their care;
- associated responsibilities/powers: this would include powers to investigate complaints, refer a case to a Mental Health Tribunal on a point of law, investigate the circumstances of a death and publish an annual report to be laid before Parliament. The inspectorate might also have a special role in advising on standards for training specialist mental health advocates.

This brief outline of the Inspectorate's functions does not mention any role in assuring the quality of training for key practitioners other than advocates. The responsibility for making appointments to the panel of experts appointed to advise the Tribunal and carry out the Second Opinion Doctor function was also removed. In fact, the safeguard that patients could not be given treatment beyond three months from the date of a tribunal order without approval from a Second Opinion Doctor was taken out of the draft Bill altogether.

The Government appeared determined to carry through the option of abolishing the MHAC and transferring its functions to a division of another regulatory body, although, only three years earlier, this was thought to be politically untenable. Besides the resource benefits, the Government identified a number of advantages in bringing together, within the Healthcare Commission, the functions of the inspection of general mental health services and the monitoring of the implementation of mental health legislation. These were:

* the new inspectorate would result in a rationalisation in the number of external regulatory bodies subjecting mental health providers to scrutiny;
* one body would be able to tackle patients' concerns about all aspects of care whether they are about legal issues, clinical quality or cleanliness;
* a new joined-up body would have more teeth and be more able to tackle identified problems.

Although not specifically asked, a number of respondents to the Mental Health Bill consultation did express reservations on the proposed organisational arrangements. A common view was that the scrutiny functions should be preserved in one specialist body, which is autonomous and free from political influence and not part of the Department of Health. The Mental Health Act Commission listed the following concerns about its demise.

i. Whether patients subject to compulsion would have a high enough priority within a general inspectorate to ensure that their interests are properly safeguarded.
ii. Whether a general inspectorate would be, or would be perceived as, having sufficient independence from Government or from the general monitoring of the NHS to provide the necessary safeguards for patients deprived of their liberty under statutory powers.
iii. Whether inspectorate visits would be sufficiently frequent to ensure that abuses could not be overlooked.
iv. Whether people with the necessary skills and expertise to monitor the implementation of mental health legislation would be attracted to work in a general healthcare inspectorate.
v. Whether responsibilities vested in a healthcare inspectorate would enable the implementation of powers exercised in relation to patients subject to compulsion by social care providers to be properly monitored. This is particularly relevant in monitoring the use of non-residential treatment orders.

It is interesting to note the contrasting position in Scotland, which moved more quickly than England in passing the Mental Health (Care and Treatment) (Scotland) Act 2003 into legislation. This legislates for the continued existence of the Scottish Mental Welfare Commission as an independent body. The Mental Welfare Commission has always had wider powers than its sister body in England, having been charged with overall protective responsibility for people with mental disorder, whether in hospital or elsewhere and is not restricted to being solely concerned with patients subject to compulsion. The new Act increases the remit of the Mental Welfare Commission still further by specifying that it should have the function of promoting best practice in as well as monitoring the operation of the Act.

Another model worthy of consideration would be for the Mental Health Act monitoring body to come under the umbrella of an Equality Body, which the Government is proposing in order to bring together the Race Equality, Equal Opportunities and Disability Commissions. Such a proposal would have all the more relevance should the new body also incorporate responsibilities for overseeing the Human Rights Act. There may also be lessons which can be learned in the field of mental health from the power which these three Commissions have to take direct action by serving notices on organisations to prescribe changes in practices or procedures or to take legal action on behalf of individuals who have been discriminated against.

A major concern of a number of respondents to the consultation on the first draft Bill was the nature of the visiting function to be carried out by the Inspectorate. The Government proposals conceded that there should be an additional safeguard for the Inspectorate to have a power to visit, but that this should be limited to where there is an identified cause for concern. It was feared that the loss of the power held by the current MHAC to visit routinely and on an unannounced basis would reduce the protection for individuals who do not seek help through other safeguards. It was argued a patient's mental disorder combined with being subject to compulsion imposes a proactive duty to visit and that it is unreasonable to expect that patients should be required to make a complaint before their concerns are addressed.

The Healthcare Commission, in its response to the first draft Bill, pointed to the advantages of a joined up body reducing the burden of inspection and, with its powers of enforcement, enabling a more systematic remedy for shortcomings. However, the scrutiny function would require a focus on individual casework not suited either to its visiting approach, which is to look at the entire system of healthcare, or the cycle of clinical governance reviews, which take place in NHS hospitals once every four years. There was also a need for there to be consistency with the independent sector, where registered mental nursing homes are subject to much more frequent inspections. Hence, the Healthcare Commission advocated that the Inspectorate should have a power to conduct regular inspections of the operation of the Mental Health Act.

However even with regular inspections, only a minority of patients are seen. The practice of the MHAC was to undertake two patient focused and one full visit in a two year visiting cycle – the purpose of the former was to concentrate on interviews with detained patients and to scrutinise the legal documents and of the latter to review the development and provision of the service overall. The MHAC estimated that, on average, Commissioners meet with about one in 15 of all detained patients and check the documentation or meet informally with a further one in six of all such patients (Ninth Biennial Report 1999-2001, p.100). The Government envisaged that the routine visiting function would be superseded by the statutory availability of advocates. The first draft Bill specified that advocacy must be made available to patients subject to compulsion and those with long term incapacity. Advocates would have a right to meet patients in private and to inspect records relating to the patient. These proposals were further articulated in the consultation document on independent specialist advocacy, published around the same time as the draft Bill.[7] It was proposed that advocates should make contact with service users within three working days of their becoming subject to the powers of the Mental Health Act and on each renewal thereafter.

It was envisaged that advocates would be a local arm of the Healthcare Commission. They would provide the first line of independent advice and support for service users who approach the Inspectorate direct with concerns, only referring back to the Healthcare Commission if they cannot deal with the issue at local level. The Healthcare Commission would provide advice to specialist advocates who are seeking guidance on aspects of the Mental Health Act and be informed by them about concerns regarding care, treatment or the operation of the Act, lending its weight to ensuring appropriate action is taken. It was thought that the Healthcare Commission would also have a role in ensuring that service users have access to the specialist advocacy service and in investigating any complaints made against a specialist advocacy service.

These proposals blurred the distinction between inspection and advocacy. The expectation that advocates might, in some way, act as agents of the inspectorate would compromise the advocacy role. That role is to help the individual get the information he or she needs to make an informed choice about what he or she wants to do without making any judgements about that choice. This will not always be compatible with the scrutiny role of the Inspectorate, which principally is to ensure that the legal requirements of compulsion are met. An advocate's authority to intervene, which must come from the service user, should not extend to examining the notes to check whether procedures have been properly carried out, if the user does not wish the advocate to become involved.

The MHAC, in its Tenth Biennial Report has conveyed its concern about the role of scrutinising the application of the Mental Health Act being diminished under the proposed arrangements. It argued that the State has an unavoidable duty to provide protection against possible breaches of human rights, which would include monitoring the use of powers of compulsion under the Mental Health Act. It referred to the judgment in the Munjaz case,[8] in which it was recognised that in

---

7   Barnes, D., Branden, T. and Webb, T. (June 2002), Independent Specialist Advocacy in England and Wales: recommendations for good practice.

8   The case involved a challenge by an Ashworth Hospital patient, who was secluded according to hospital policy which did not comply with Code of Practice guidance. The Court of Appeal ruled that guidance in the Code must be observed unless there is good reason for departing from it in relation to individual patients. The judgment was overruled by the House

cases "where the state itself has deprived a vulnerable person his liberty and the state itself is responsible for how that person is treated. … the state ought to know enough about its own prisoner or patient to provide effective protection from inhuman or degrading treatment …" In order to protect the scrutinising function, the MHAC has recommended that there should be an explicit requirement within a new Act for the Secretary of State to provide for the monitoring and review of powers and duties as they relate to the compulsion of patients. The credibility of this scrutiny function would depend, in the MHAC view, on the retention of the power to visit on a regular basis. Such visiting would need to be of sufficient frequency to ensure that abuse and poor practice is not overlooked.

The Government appeared to have been swayed by these arguments. The second draft Bill, published in September 2004, separated the roles of an inspectorate and advocacy. The role of the Independent Mental Health Advocate would be more narrowly circumscribed and was outlined as including:

- help in obtaining information about the medical treatment being provided to the patient;
- information about why the treatment is being provided;
- information about the legal authority under which the patient is being treated;
- advice about the patient's rights, including the right to apply for discharge.

The advocate would have the right to meet the patient, but access to the patient's records would be subject to veto by hospital managers, who must have regard to any wishes and feelings expressed by the patient about such access. The Government accepted that a more proactive visiting regime on the part of the Healthcare Commission was a necessary safeguard in addition to and separate from the involvement of an advocate. The Commission would not only have the power to visit where there was a particular cause for concern, but would also be able to do so as a preventative measure on a programmed or random basis. Thus it would retain similar powers to the MHAC to visit and meet with patients subject to compulsion, including the right to make unannounced visits. However, there is no specification concerning the frequency of visits, only that the Healthcare Commission should undertake investigations, if it thinks it necessary or expedient to do so.

The Richardson Committee recommended that there should be a successor body to the MHAC, fully independent of State agencies and of Government, which should be answerable directly to Parliament. Through the various stages in the consultation process on the reform of the Mental Health Act, the successor body was reduced to a division of a new Health Care Inspectorate. How much does this downgrading of status matter?

---

of Lords (R vs Ashworth Hospital Authority ex parte Munjaz [2005] UKHL 58). It referred to the Code's introduction, which states that there is no legal duty to comply with it, but that it is a statutory document and failure to follow it could be referred to in evidence in legal proceedings.

A number of scrutiny functions can be performed by other bodies, notably the new Mental Health Tribunal and specialist advocacy services. Compulsion which continues beyond 28 days must be sanctioned by an independent tribunal, who will also have to be satisfied that an appropriate care plan is in place. The tribunal will have access to a panel of experts, consisting of medical and other specialists. These independent experts will interview and examine the patient in private and inspect any records relating to the patient and then must prepare a report for the tribunal. Their role, as does that of the current Second Opinion Appointed Doctor, could incorporate a check to confirm that the statutory detention documentation is in order. The statutory right to specialist advocacy services should enable every patient to have speedy access to independent advice about their legal position and rights. Potentially, it provides a more effective safeguard than MHAC visits, the periodic nature of which has meant that most patients do not have an opportunity to see a Commissioner. Local advocates could support service users who wish to make a complaint. Indeed, the MHAC's complaints remit has already been largely superseded by the revamped NHS complaints procedures.

Despite its weak remit and lack of resources, the MHAC has improved professional and institutional practice in the implementation of the Act and the care and treatment of detained patients. Undoubtedly, it could have done more. There have been a number of reports condemning the standards of in-patient care.[9] In a briefing note released in June 2002, the Sainsbury Centre for Mental Health has warned that the situation is little short of a crisis with the quality of care in adult acute psychiatric in-patient care so poor in some instances as to amount to a basic denial of human rights. The MHAC's regular visiting has failed to ensure that good or even adequate quality care is provided in units where patients are liable to be detained.

Over recent years, during the crucial period of consultation on the reform of the Mental Health Act, the MHAC went through a period of instability. It lacked leadership and its influence waned. The Government's proposals to abolish the MHAC and replace it with a Mental Health Act division of a new Health Care Inspectorate will further reduce any influence. No reference was made to the MHAC, for example, in the Healthcare Commission's sector report on what that body had found in its inspections of mental health trusts. This report was published at the same time as the MHAC's Tenth Report[10] in December 2003 and raised similar concerns

---

9   Gourney, K., Ward, M., Thornicroft, G. and Wright, S. (1998), 'Crisis in the capital: inpatient care in inner London', *Mental Health Practice*, 1(5), 10-18.

Sainsbury Centre for Mental Health (1998), *Acute Problems: A survey of the quality of care in acute psychiatric wards*, London: The Sainsbury Centre for Mental Health.

DoH (1999), *Mental Health Nursing Addressing Acute Concerns*, Report of the Standing Nursing and Midwifery Advisory Committee.

DoH (2002), *Mental Health Policy Implementation Guide*, Adult Acute Inpatient Care Provision.

Commission for Health Improvement (undated), *What CHI has found in mental health trusts*, Sector Report.

10 The Mental Health Act Commission (2003), Tenth Biennial Report 2001-2003, *Placed amongst strangers. Twenty years of the Mental Health Act 1983 and future prospects for compulsion*, London: TSO.

about severe pressures on adult acute in-patient units, the safety of patients, the restrictions on the liberty of informal patients and the lack of compliance with Code of Practice standards in the use of seclusion. However, in 2004, a concordat was agreed between bodies inspecting, regulating and auditing healthcare, which aims to achieve grater consistency and cohesion in the inspection process.

The Government announced its intention within the 2005 budget proposals, as part of its policy to reduce the number of arm's length bodies, to merge the Healthcare and Care Standards Commissions into a much larger body. The Joint Parliamentary Committee on the Draft Mental Health Bill regarded it as almost inevitable that the functions to scrutinise the operation of mental health legislation would become diluted within such a large organisation. In the Joint Committee's view,

> It is vital that, if the monitoring of compulsory powers is to be effective, patients know who is doing it and how they are doing it. This is more likely to be the case if there is a focused stand-alone body with a high profile and clear title.[11]

---

11 House of Lords and House of Commons Joint Committee on the Draft Mental Health Bill, Vol. 1, p.108.

Index